GERD Diet:

The Complete and Effective GERD Diet Easy Meal Plan with Delicious Recipes & Proven Natural Remedies for the Relief of GERD

Daniel Michaels

© Copyright 2018 by Daniel Michaels - All rights reserved.

The contents of this book may not be reproduced, duplicated or transmitted without direct written permission from the author.

Under no circumstances will any legal responsibility or blame be held against the publisher for any reparation, damages, or monetary loss due to the information herein, either directly or indirectly.

Legal Notice:

This book is copyright protected. This is only for personal use. You cannot amend, distribute, sell, use, quote or paraphrase any part or the content within this book without the consent of the author.

Disclaimer Notice:

Please note the information contained within this document is for educational and entertainment purposes only. Every attempt has been made to provide accurate, up to date and reliable complete information. No warranties of any kind are expressed or implied. Readers acknowledge that the author is not engaging in the rendering of legal, financial, medical or professional advice. The content of this book has been derived from various sources. Please consult a licensed professional before attempting any techniques outlined in this book.

By reading this document, the reader agrees that under no circumstances are is the author responsible for any losses, direct or indirect, which are incurred as a result of the use of information contained within this document, including, but not limited to, —errors, omissions, or inaccuracies.

Table of Contents

Introduction

Chapter 1: GERD – Knowing the Essentials

Chapter 2: The Natural Remedies for GERD

Chapter 3: The GERD Diet Meal Plan

Chapter 4: Breakfast

Chapter 5: Soups

Chapter 6: Salads

Chapter 7: Snacks

Chapter 8: Lunch

Chapter 9: Dinner

Chapter 10: Desserts

BONUS Chapter: GERD Diet for

Weight Loss

Conclusion

What This Book Will Teach You

Are you currently suffering from GERD and looking for natural remedy solutions but unsure where to start?

Have you always wanted to cure your GERD symptoms, but want to have a comprehensive reference on how to help treat it?

If these questions relate well with you, then this book is for you. In this book, you will discover all about GERD and the natural methods for healing. This book also introduces the reader to the GERD Diet Meal Plan, and the delicious recipes that one can prepare for a healthier lifestyle.

Who this Book is for

This book contains information on an effective GERD diet that can help relieve them of their GERD symptoms.

Readers who can benefit the most from the book include:

- GERD sufferers who want to know alternative methods on how to help relieve symptoms

- Readers who want to learn about the GERD diet and meal plan as an alternative solution to treating GERD symptoms.

How this Book is Organized

This book is organized into three parts. The parts are best read in chronological order. Once you become familiar with all the steps outlined in the book, you can go directly to the techniques which apply to your current situation the best.

The three parts of the book are:

Part One outlines the essential topics

on GERD. The section also talks about how important it is to learn these topics as a beginner in order to form a solid foundation in doing the right steps – from introductory concepts to preparing your first healthy meal.

Part Two is about the GERD Diet Meal Plan and what one can do to implement it for a healthier lifestyle. You'll learn how the process works and how to implement the steps discussed.

Part Three are the healthy recipes you can prepare. It also has a Bonus Chapter on Weight Loss.

Introduction:

Thank you for owning this book on GERD Diet: The Complete and Effective GERD Diet Easy Meal Plan with Delicious Recipes & Proven Natural Remedies for the Relief of GERD and I hope that it is able to provide you with all the help that you need for alleviating and healing your GERD problem.

In this book, we will discuss what you need to know about GERD, how it is diagnosed, and what you can do to naturally and effectively heal it. We talk about the symptoms that you can expect when dealing with GERD. We discuss how Doctors diagnose GERD and what types of medical treatments there are. Then we talk about the natural ways that we can treat GERD. Although there are many treatment options, the most effective way to deal with any health condition is to treat the underlying problems and with GERD, that is your diet.

This book will also walk you through on what you can and cannot eat with GERD. We explain how food affects you and how without the proper diet you can cause more severe GERD issues. We also go into detail on what other conditions can come about by not properly treating your GERD.

This book, is not only, geared to help you understand what GERD is, but how you yourself can treat your GERD at home, with natural remedies that do not have harmful side effects. Many medications for GERD have some severe and harmful side effects. Some of those side effects can be heart disease, stomach poisoning, and nutritional deficiencies that can ultimately harm you. Another condition, that can come from not properly treating your GERD, is pre-cancerous lesions, called Barrett's esophagus.

I hope you enjoy this book and the recipes that we have included for you to utilize to help heal your GERD. Food is a natural healer and when we use it properly without processing and added chemicals we can begin to heal our lives. Each chapter has helpful, and educational material that will not only bring you closer to understanding your condition but also will help you with some steps to take to alleviate and heal your gut.

Chapter 1: GERD - Knowing the Essentials

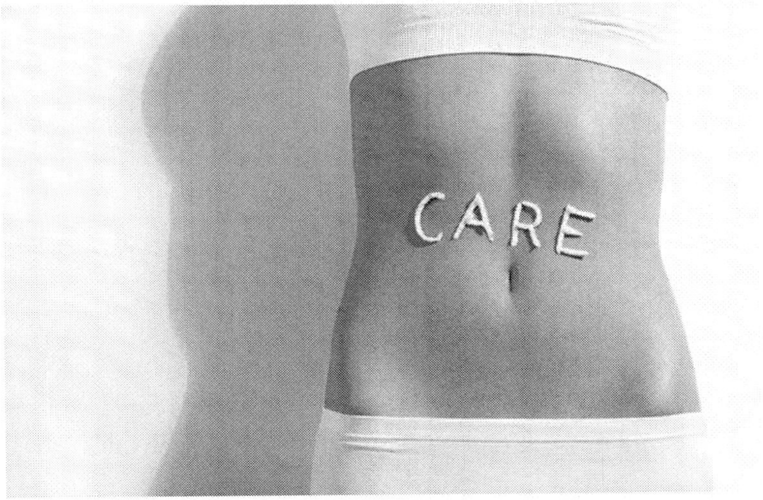
CARE

Chapter 1: GERD – Knowing the Essentials

What is GERD and what should you know about it?

GERD or Gastroesophageal reflux disease, is a digestive ailment. It affects your lower esophageal sphincter. This is the ring of muscles that separate the esophagus and the stomach. There are many people who suffer from GERD. GERD can be caused by a hiatal hernia and dietary issues. If you adjust your diet you can begin to change your GERD, however sometimes in more severe cases, you will need medications and even surgery.

When suffering from GERD, your lower esophageal sphincter is too weak to block out the stomach contents. This allows the stomach contents to flow up into your esophagus. This also takes place when the lower sphincter is too relaxed, causing the same reflux of stomach contents.

Although many people think GERD is the same thing as Acid Reflux, it is similar but not the same. GERD happens when the Lower Esophageal is weakened, but acid reflux is the backflow of stomach acid. In GERD, your stomach contents are coming back through the sphincter, however, in acid reflux, the stomach acid backflows or regurgitates into your throat.

What symptoms do you experience during GERD?

With acid reflux you will experience sour liquid in your throat, you may taste some regurgitated food, and feel a burning sensation in your chest, such as heartburn. In GERD you experience many different symptoms. Some of those symptoms are a heavy chest or difficulty breathing due to the heartburn. You may also experience a lump or knot in your throat as if your food has not gone down to your stomach. Another thing you may also experience is decaying teeth.

This is a result of the acid flowing up into your mouth and a sour bitter taste. Some people experience difficulty swallowing, and a hoarse voice or coughing. These can be accompanied by a sore throat. Although these are just some of the symptoms that separate GERD from acid reflux, there are several more differences. Many people intermingle acid reflux and heartburn with GERD, however, they are clearly different conditions. Heartburn is just the symptom of acid reflux and GERD. GERD is a long-term, more serious, chronic condition that several people suffer from.

So what causes GERD to happen?

The simple answer, most of our diets are not good for our stomachs. We eat too many spicy foods, drink caffeine and alcohol in excess, and eat way too much chocolate, peppermint, fried foods, fatty foods, and foods heavy with sauce. All of these foods can aggravate and irritate the esophageal sphincter and result in GERD symptoms. Many women develop GERD during pregnancy, and smokers have more relaxed lower esophageal sphincters. Another factor can be weight, such as obesity.

Some of the most common symptoms of GERD include heartburn. Heartburn starts as a burning sensation, or pressure that feels painful. It can feel like your food is coming back up into your throat. Episodes can last as little as 2 hours. Often times it is brought on by bending, lying down, or after eating. Mixing spicy foods, alcohol, and ibuprofen can cause your GERD to act up, resulting in several of the symptoms of GERD.

A diagnosis of GERD is only right about 70% of the time. It presents with many similar symptoms as other acid reflux type conditions and can be misdiagnosed due to no known testing process. When testing for GERD the doctor should check into the history of nausea, vomiting, or regurgitate. This could be signs of a delayed gastric emptying. People with GERD can experience other conditions that are associated with GERD. Some of these can include complications such as esophagitis, stricture, and Barrett's esophagus. Doctors estimate that 50% of GERD suffers will develop esophagitis.

Reflux is one of the most common causes of chest pain. If myocardial infarction is ruled out, then you are experiencing GERD and the normal procedure would be to administer a high-dose proton pump inhibitor or PPI. People that present with these symptoms are atypical for many GERD sufferers. They can additionally experience damage to their lungs due to the acid. Other damages can include vocal cords and ear and teeth, issues.

GERD has two main forms, one that is Non-erosive, and one that is Erosive. Most people who suffer from GERD suffer from the Non-erosive form, NERD. The main concern with patients who suffer from GERD is developing Barrett's esophagus, also known as a pre-cancerous lesion. The natural progression of GERD has been found to start with Non-erosive that progresses to mild Erosive. However, mild Erosive can progress to severely Erosive and then, in turn, progresses further to Barrett's esophagus. Barrett's esophagus is likely to happen in only about 1% to 13% of patients who suffer from GERD.

Learning more about GERD can help you handle your conditions.

So how do you deal with your GERD? Knowing how to deal with your GERD is an important part of maintaining your health. Although GERD is totally manageable, many people do not manage their diet and essentially cause themselves more complications.

You should be well informed of what not to eat so that you do not aggravate your GERD. Knowing what not to eat is the first step in being prepared for maintaining your GERD. GERD can be quite painful at times and knowing how to manage your diet will keep you from experiencing symptoms.

Knowing how to handle your GERD can also prevent it from progressing. When

GERD progresses, it can cause many other complications. Maintaining your diet and treatments can help reduce the reflux and damage that is being caused to your lining of the esophagus. By avoiding foods and beverages that can cause inflammation of your GERD you can prevent further damage. Some of those foods are:

- Chocolate
- Peppermint
- Alcohol
- Fatty foods
- Coffee
- Spicy food
- Garlic
- Onions
- Citrus foods
- And juices
- As well as tomato products

- And pepper

Other foods contribute to your GERD symptoms, and these should be avoided as much as possible. When we are more informed about our dietary needs and how to manage our GERD, we can better handle the symptoms that come along with GERD.

By maintaining your diet and medications regimen you will receive the benefits of:

- Less acid reflux
- A reduced chance of getting Barrett's esophagus
- Reduce your painful heartburn and irritated throat
- Have a healthier diet
- And feel better in general.

How do we diagnose GERD?

Diagnosing GERD is not based on a medical test. It is basically diagnosed through an extensive intake of your symptoms and conditions. The doctor will start by asking you some questions about your symptoms and how long you have been experiencing them.

He may start with any number of tests to verify you have GERD.

- Medication to quantify if it is GERD, by seeing if the medication reduces the symptoms.
- An ambulatory acid probe helps them determine the pH of acid found in your esophagus.
- An endoscopy of your upper respiratory can determine if you are at risk for ulcers.

- If the patient is showing conditions similar to Barrett's esophagus, then the Doctor may order regular endoscopy procedures.

CHAPTER SUMMARY:

1.1 We discussed what GERD is and how you can identify the symptoms that are associated with GERD. We talked about how acid reflux and GERD are two different disorders and the differences between the two. We then talked about how to know the difference between GERD and heart attack, since they have similar pain symptoms in your chest.

1.2 We discussed some of the symptoms that come with GERD and what you as a patient can expect. We discussed what causes GERD and some historical information on how GERD affects your body and how it progresses over time.

1.3 We then discuss why it is important to learn more about GERD. The types of foods to avoid and why it's important to avoid them. We also talked about how the Doctor will diagnose GERD. The methods he will use to diagnose and monitor your GERD progress.

YOUR QUICK START ACTION STEP:

We are all concerned with our health. One way to be more vigilant with your health knowledge is to check out more information on symptoms and treatments that will help maintain your GERD.

Chapter 2: The Natural Remedies for GERD

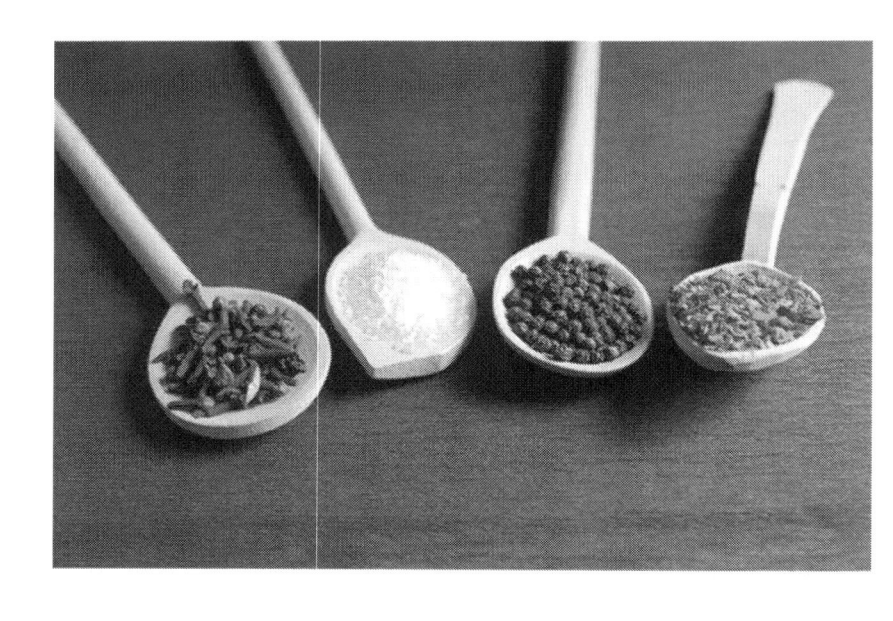

Chapter 2: The Natural Remedies for GERD

In the previous chapter, we talked about what GERD is and the many ways it can unfortunately affect your life. We also talked about the differences between GERD and acid reflux. We have discussed how to diagnose GERD and how to maintain your health while having GERD. We also discussed the history of GERD and how it can progress into a much more serious pre-cancerous condition. In this chapter, we will discuss the natural remedies that can be used to treat and alleviate symptoms of GERD. We will discuss how each remedy is effective and why it is effective. We also talk about how to use the remedy, or how to incorporate it into your life.

GERD is just like most other conditions that people struggle with in that it is not an issue that you have to deal with at face value. It can be alleviated and maintained when using a proper diet and medication routine. However, there are several natural remedies that will prevent you from having to use medications for maintenance of your GERD. You will need to be diligent in your fight, however, as it is not something that will improve on its own.

Natural remedies can consist of supplements, and a proper diet, as well as, exercise. Although natural remedies can be a wide range of things, they are usually your best option for taking care of your health. In this chapter, we go over several suggestions that you can incorporate into your life, without too much change to your current lifestyle. As with any natural remedy, we want to make sure it will not be contraindicative to any other conditions that you have, as well as medications you are already taking. You want to ensure that it will not harm you, due to any of your current medications. As always, speak with your Doctor before adding anything new to your health plan. What natural remedies can you use to treat or alleviate GERD?

Baking Soda

Many people are finding that baking soda is a natural remedy for treating GERD due to its ability to neutralize the acid. It can be used effectively for short time periods and should be used no more than seven times in one day. The basic recipe, for a baking soda neutralizing drink, is to place 1 tsp into an 8-oz. glass of water and drink it up to seven times per day. However, you do not want to use it for more than a week. This method can be effective in neutralizing the acid in your stomach and in the event that the acid comes up, it will be less painful due to no acid burns. It does contain a high content of salt though, so It is best to not use it more than recommended and it can, in fact, cause swelling and upset stomach.

Remain upright after eating

Although this should be common sense, it is not a good idea to lay down within 4 hours of eating. However, many people still eat and then lay down, without thinking about digesting their food first. This is one of the worst things you can do for your body, especially if you have

GERD. When you eat food and then lie flat, it allows the contents of your stomach to be easily brought back up your esophagus. The sphincter is relaxed causing acid reflux. Staying upright can prevent a good bit of this complication. It allows gravity to work for you, by keeping the stomach contents in the stomach. By eating a few hours before going to bed, at least 4, you are giving yourself a better chance of not having any symptoms. Sleeping elevated can help this process also.

Ginger Tea

Ginger is a great stomach aid. It not only alleviates stomach upset, and nausea, but also symptoms of GERD. To get the best benefit of ginger tea, you should slice some ginger root and place it into a pot of water that has boiled for 30 minutes. Let the ginger root seep in the water, allowing the flavor to set in. For best results, drink your tea before dinner, this will help reduce the acid that will be produced.

Chamomile Tea

To help balance your acidity levels in your stomach, use chamomile tea for 30 minutes before bedtime. Chamomile has been known to reduce stress levels, which is a big contributor to GERD and acid reflux. Making chamomile tea is a simple process and you can make it fresh or buy an already blended tea. Let the chamomile seep for 45 minutes before drinking it. Chamomile is also a great relaxant that will help you sleep as well.

Chewing Gum

Studies have shown that chewing sugar-free gum for 30 minutes can alleviate GERD by increasing your saliva. With increased saliva, you can alleviate the acid that is in your mouth. The saliva will wash away the acid making it less likely for you to experience GERD symptoms. Chew your sugar-free gum right after your meal to help reduce the effects of the acid reflux.

Follow a GERD diet

Many people have had tremendous success treating their GERD through a proper GERD diet. The first thing you should do is stop eating inflammatory foods. You should adjust your diet to include anti-inflammatory foods. There are several foods that create sensitivities in those with GERD, such as gluten, dairy, and processed foods with synthetic ingredients. Several foods make pain worse, such as:

- Caffeine
- Chocolate
- Alcohol
- High-sodium foods
- Garlic
- Tomatoes
- Onions
- Mint
- Citrus food
- Fatty foods
- Refined grains
- Spicy foods

Instead eat foods that are fresh, such as, fresh vegetables, grass-fed lean meats, nuts, seeds, healthy fats, coconut oil, apples, berries, pears, bone broth, and yogurt. Other things that you can limit in your diet would be carbonated drinks. As well as limiting your diet, you should eat smaller meals. You will need 5 small meals a day instead of three large meals a day. This helps you process the food easier and reduces the chances of GERD inflammation. You should also eat slower, and drink slower. This helps you chew slower and reduces your acid levels. Avoid using straws and smoking. These can cause you to take in more air and create air bubbles. When the air enters the digestive system, it can inflame your GERD.

Avoid wearing tight clothes

Tight clothing restricts your ability to breathe and also restricts your digestion. It is more difficult to be comfortable and digest your food if your stomach is in tight clothes. By restricting your digestive track, you are creating inflammation and blocking your food from processing.

Drink more water

By drinking more water, you can lower your symptoms of GERD. Water can replace caffeine, sugary drinks, and alcohol. When you drink more water, you are hydrating your body and eliminating the inflammation in your stomach.

Manage your stress and get more rest

By managing your stress, you are able to

lower your GERD symptoms. Try relaxing more, getting more exercise, and meditating. All of these can help you manage your stress and also helps you get more rest. When your body is well rested, and you are less stressed your stomach will be less inflamed and you will have fewer issues with GERD and stomach acid.

Quit Smoking

Smoking can cause your esophagus sphincter to be relaxed and create symptoms of GERD. By quitting you can alleviate your GERD symptoms and help your body to heal. GERD can be agitated by smoking, so the sooner you stop the better.

Maintain a healthy weight and get more exercise

Research has proven that obesity is a natural cause of GERD. By being sedentary and consuming more processed, unhealthy food items, you are causing inflammation in your stomach on a regular basis. When you eat a healthy diet and get more exercise you can balance your hormones and reduce your inflammation, which in turn reduces your GERD.

Licorice

Deglycyrrhizinated licorice root, otherwise known as licorice, has been found to be an effective acid reflux treatment. You can chew 2 tablets, 20 minutes before every meal, 3 times per day, or you can take it right before bed to prevent suffering during the night. Make sure you use only the chewable DCL because it must be combined with your saliva so that you get the results that you need. A great one to use is one by Enzymatic Therapy.

Probiotics

Probiotics introduce micro-organisms into the stomach that helps neutralize toxic compounds in the stomach. Although you can purchase a supplement in the grocery store, a better option is to buy fermented vegetables, kefir, and fermented, unpasteurized beer. You can also use fermented milk products, such as buttermilk, clabber, cheese, and yogurt. Another great option is fermented soy products such as natto, tempeh, soy sauce, miso, and fermented tofu. You should include these on a regular basis in your diet. They will help correct your acid reflux problems.

D-Limonene Extract

The d-limonene extract is an extract from citrus peel. It provides a protective coating for the stomach and esophagus. Although there is no scientific explanation of why this works, there have been trials to show that it actually does provide relief. In said trial, the participants took one gram of D-Limonene every 20 days and after two weeks 90% of them had experienced relief. And after a single treatment program, they had relief from GERD which lasted up to 6 months.

Herbs that treat or alleviate GERD

There are several herbs that can alleviate and even treat GERD. Although peppermint is an inflammatory, using peppermint oil can alleviate GERD, along with other herbs listed below:

- Ginger Root
- Caraway
- Garden angelica
- German chamomile flower
- Greater celandine
- Licorice root
- Lemon balm
- Milk thistle
- Turmeric

All of these herbs can be found in health food stores and can be cost effective for treating GERD. You can use them as teas, oils and even capsules. Herbs have no government regulations so make sure you research what you can take with your current health conditions and medications. Several herbs cannot be mixed together, so make sure you follow the instructions perfectly.

Antioxidants

Vitamins rich in A, C, and E are being used effectively to prevent GERD. Most of the time these vitamin supplements are only used to add nutrients your body is lacking. A blood test, done by your doctor, can determine what you are lacking so that you can get the right supplements. Some doctors may even suggest a multi-vitamin.

Melatonin

Melatonin is a sleep hormone that is found naturally in your body. It is also a supplement that you can purchase in pill form at the grocery store. Using melatonin for sleep is a natural remedy; however, studies have shown that using melatonin for GERD is effective. Melatonin is produced in the pineal gland, which is located in your brain. Through some preliminary studies, they have found that due to melatonin's ability to relax the mind, it also has a long-term relief for GERD symptoms. However, you must combine it with another form of reflux treatment, due to it not working on its own.

Why should you use natural remedies instead of medication?

Although medication is effective for treating GERD, it can carry some pretty serious side effects. So instead of using medication, you can effectively treat your GERD through natural remedies.

Natural remedies provide you a safe alternative to traditional medication. As a society, we have been so dependent on medications, that we have lost sight of how to properly care for our bodies. Although GERD can be caused by pregnancy or other health-related conditions, it is widely caused by obesity. By making your health better you can essentially make your gut better, which will alleviate your GERD. Often times you will hear, if you heal your gut you can heal your body. This is so true. When we heal our gut, we start to heal all the other medical conditions that we have been living with. Doctors have found that our gut contributes to most of our health-related issues. Based on the food that we take in, this determines the nutrients, vitamins, and minerals that our body processes. If we are only eating junk and processed foods, then our body is not getting proper care. Then we start to develop medical conditions, not understanding why we are sick.

Natural remedies can also save you money. The medical remedies to GERD tend to be expensive. They can cost lots of money that your insurance may not pay for. So instead of spending lots of money on medications that will cause side effects, start trying the natural remedies that we have listed here in this chapter. Many of the natural remedies that are listed above below include changing your diet, which is a big part of healing your gut. Start with changing your diet and then move on to making more drastic and powerful changes that can effectively heal your GERD, without the high cost of medication.

What benefits do you receive from using natural remedies as opposed to medical treatments?

Benefits of using natural remedies

- By changing your diet, you can reduce your grocery expense.

- If you are eating heathy you feel more energized.

- That extra energy allows you to get more exercise.

- Essentially allowing you to be healthier and have less stress.

- When you have less stress, you can get more sleep.

- Sleeping more helps the body heal faster.

- Your body reacts to positive

health habits and starts to heal your GERD.

- By not eating, within 4 hours of laying down, you can reduce your risk of having symptoms. This also helps you to digest your food properly.

- Using herbal remedies decreases your need for medications such as PPI's, which listed below can create more problems than they help.

- By reducing your food in-take, you can prevent from over eating, which is a leading cause of acid reflux.

- By changing what you eat and how you eat, you can eliminate the inflammatory intake of foods that cause the reflux.

- Cutting back on alcohol, caffeine and spicy foods, will get rid of the heartburn all together, eliminating your chances of damaging your esophagus.

- Doctors recommend trying all the other natural remedies before going to medications. Due to their side effects, and how harmful they can be.

Medical disadvantages

- Medicine can cost more money than food and natural remedies.

- It can have side effects that will cause you to need more medicines.

- They can be less effective.

- Medicine can also cause more weight gain.

- Which causes more GERD.

- They do not address the cause of the GERD which is a permanent damage to the lower esophageal sphincter.

- Your episodes of reflux will not decrease by taking medications. It has been proven that they do not stop or limit the number of acidic episodes.

- The medications will not prevent the development of Barrett's esophagus.

- Every single acid suppressant has side effects. These side effects can be significant when used on a long-term basis. Due to the acid suppressing effects of these medications, it is not only, suppressing the over active acid that causes the concern, but also the acid used to digest properly.

There are many health risks associated with the suppression of acid:

.1 Increased risk of pneumonia

.2 Chronic kidney disease

.3 E. coli infections

.4 Stroke

.5 Heart attacks

.6 Calcium malabsorption

.7 Increase in clostridium difficile infections, which is a digestive system infection that is life threatening.

.8 Campylobacter enteritis increase

.9 Increased risk of hospitalization for infectious gastroenteritis

- The acid reflux medications should be used no longer than 2 weeks at a time.

- Knowledge of these drugs is key to making them work, however, losing weight and proper diet are paramount to healing.

- PPI's leave you vulnerable to nutritional deficiencies and infections.

- Increased risk of food poisoning due to improper digestion, because of the lack of acid.

- Because PPI's stop the production of stomach acid, it becomes increasingly harder to digest your food, block the intake of proper vitamins, nutrients, and minerals needed to be healthy.

- This includes nutrients for helping keep the bones strong.
- As well as an increase in your chances of dementia

Recipe and instruction on using one natural remedy for treatment.

Turmeric is a natural remedy for treating acid reflux. We discussed above a few herbs that can help alleviate or treat GERD. In this section, we will give you a step by step instruction guide on using turmeric for acid reflux.

Turmeric Ginger Smoothie

Turmeric is an anti-inflammatory, and

antioxidant that helps alleviate GERD symptoms. Ginger is aids in alleviating stomach upset and nausea. In this smoothie, they have included carrot juice, strawberries, yogurt, and bananas, due to their potassium.

This recipe makes 2 servings

- Calories: 114
- Sodium 63 mg

What's In It

- Ginger (0.50tsp)
- Turmeric (1tsp)
- Ripe Banana (1 med.)
- Yogurt (4.0-oz. or 1 small cup)
- Chilled carrot juice(2c.)

How it's made

1. Start by placing all ingredients into a blender.

2. Turn the blender on and pulse it for 30 seconds until it is smooth.

3. Pour into two separate glasses and enjoy for breakfast, lunch, or snack.

CHAPTER SUMMARY:

2.1 We discussed what natural remedies you can use for your GERD, how they are effective, and why they are effective. We discuss the comparisons of medication to natural remedies and how they can be beneficial or damaging.

2.2 We talked about how the medications can affect your health and what doctors suggest would be a more viable option for treating GERD. We talk about how the natural remedies will better manage the GERD without side effects. Then we discussed how the medications can further complicate your health and how the Doctors would rather you change your lifestyle and diet before trying any medications.

2.3 Lastly, we discussed a recipe for a turmeric ginger smoothie that can be used to alleviate the symptoms. We provided information on why this smoothie is effective and the nutritional facts for the smoothie. We also talked about when it is best used.

YOUR QUICK START ACTION STEP:

One way to learn more about natural remedies that help your GERD is to do some research on your own. There are several websites that could help you with your research. Below we have listed one that is quite beneficial to those suffering from GERD.

Chapter 3: The GERD Diet Meal Plan

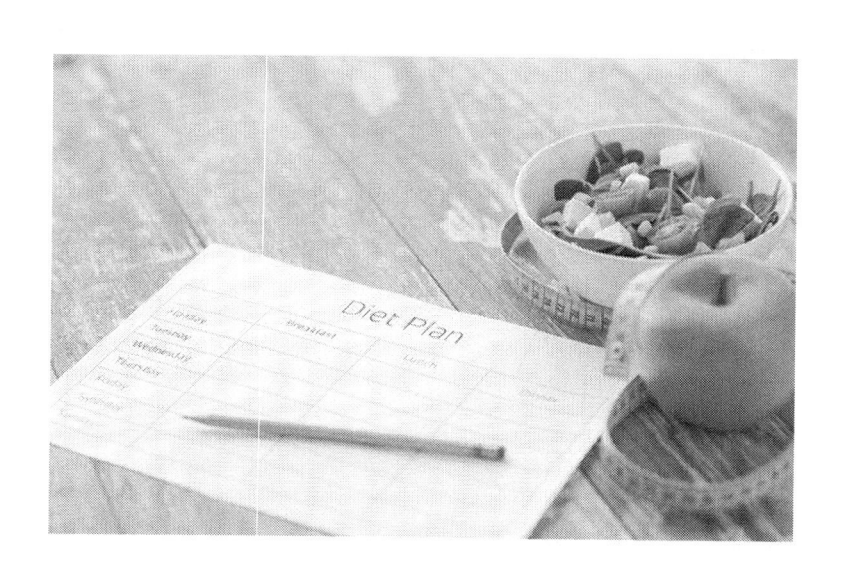

Chapter 3: GERD Diet Meal Plan

Now that we have dedicated the first chapter to what GERD is and how to tell if you have GERD. The diagnostic test that is performed by your Doctor to determine if you have GERD, and what treatments there are for it. Then we discussed natural remedies that can be utilized to alleviate the symptoms of GERD or eliminate altogether. Next, we talked about how the Doctors are finding that the medications that treat GERD are causing more damage than helping and how it is best to change your diet and lifestyle in order to get your GERD under control.

This next few chapters will be all about

discussing a GERD diet meal plan. As with any meal plan, make sure you can eat all the ingredients listed in the recipes. Check with your Doctor to make sure you are okay to start a new diet plan, as well as how it can affect you with your current medications. GERD is a disorder that deals with your stomach acid levels. When we eat a GERD approved diet we can start to lower the inflammation and reduce our symptoms, eventually correcting the disorder altogether.

One of the diet plans we will examine in this chapter is the Acid Reflux Diet. What this means is that it is a diet designed to eliminate acid reflux. This acid reflux diet is called the Pritikin Program. The Pritikin Program is designed to help you eat healthily, exercise regularly, and reduce stress. This diet will help reduce your stress and prevent any types of cardiovascular disease. Cardiovascular-related disease treatment is a solution for acid reflux and GERD.

The basic guidelines of the Pritikin Diet Program have the following key lifestyle changes.

- Exercise regularly
- Start reducing your stress by developing skills to handle stress. These skills could be meditation, yoga, and 10 minutes of deep breathing. These skills can be beneficial in so many ways.
- Make sure you get a full night sleep, every night. Lack of sleep is

a leading cause of stress and illness.
- Get plenty of whole fresh foods. Foods naturally low in fat, and sugar. These can be whole grains, fruits, nonfat dairy, vegetables, and fish.
- Stay away from fatty type meats and soft drinks, and sugary drinks. Carbonated drinks are not a good option when dealing with GERD. As well as, processed foods, sugary desserts, and fatty, fried foods.
- Do not eat spicy foods or high in acid fruits. This can be anything from oranges, to tomatoes, as well as, lemons.
- Keep a journal of all your eating patterns and when you feel your GERD being inflamed. This will

help you keep track of your triggers and symptoms. This gives you a list to work with for eliminating foods and drinks.

- Make sure you eat your dinner before 7 pm. This will guarantee that you have plenty of time to digest food before going to bed.
- Do not lie down after eating. Sit upright for several hours prior to laying down or going to bed. Another option is to take an after-dinner walk, this will help digestion, as well as prevent you from falling asleep before your food is digested. It will also help you walk off the extra lbs. you have.
- Stop smoking. Not only for your GERD but for overall health improvement.

- If you are dealing with excess weight, then consider changing your diet and exercise routine. A healthy diet can make a big difference in your GERD symptoms, as well as an exercise routine that helps burn calories and fat.

Over the next few chapters, we will be giving you recipes that will help you with your GERD diet plan. You will find 5-10 recipes for each chapter, plus at least 1-2 more complex recipes to utilize in your GERD diet meal plan. These meals can be integrated into your lifestyle by slowly adding in one GERD friendly meal a day, eliminating sugary drinks, and caffeine. By adding in one meal a day you can over time start to have all 5 small meals, as GERD friendly meals, and start to see changes in your GERD symptoms, as well as, your weight and health.

We will start our GERD diet meal plan with breakfast options. These will be low-volume meals that can reduce the pressure in your abdomen.

We will choose foods low in fat, acid and other triggers that tend to inflame you GERD. We want to start our day without inflammation, so choosing ingredients a that are low acid, and clean will help with this. Even though breakfast is you first start to the day, you still want to practice moderation and only eat small meals. This will help you digest your food easier and then allow for a mid-morning snack. Each section will have easy recipes that you can use to follow a GERD friendly diet and one more complex recipe at the end.

We will also discuss some soups and salads that are great for the GERD diet as well as several snack options that will not cause any excess acid to build up and overflow. Soups and salads are staples for most family meals. In these chapters, we will make sure they are ones that can be used in the GERD as well as providing a tremendous number of vitamins, nutrients, and minerals. The snacks section will be designed to help you choose healthy snacks that will not only satisfy those snack cravings but will be low-acidic for the GERD diet.

We will next work on lunch meals that can be used midday to help fuel you for the rest of your day. Keeping low-volume meals during lunch as well is key to maintaining the diet. One way to do this is to prepare a nutrient-rich meal and eat half of the meal at lunchtime and the other half at as a mid-afternoon snack. This will keep you energized through the day, and also allow you to maintain your acid reflux symptoms. In this chapter, we will include several easy to prepare recipes and a few more complex recipes so that you have a wide range of options to choose from.

Finally, we will discuss the best options for dinner. Although dinner is usually the biggest meal of the day, with the GERD diet we would want to make this one the lightest meal of the day. We want to get the majority of your nutrients and food intake earlier in the day. This allows for the denser ingredients to have already digested before bedtime. When we eat heavy meals late at night we tend to hold on to that fat and calorie intake much longer. So, the best way to eliminate the excess fat and reduce the symptoms of GERD is to eat earlier in the evening, do some light exercise, such as a walk after dinner, and save your nutrient-rich foods throughout the day.

This GERD Diet Meal Plan can help cure or alleviate your GERD symptoms and condition. Although, it's not a "magic cure-all" it can help you with your GERD and over time by following the diet you can eliminate the GERD conditions altogether. Curing your gut and becoming a much healthier individual.

The first step to following the GERD Diet Meal Plan is to know what you cannot have. So, we have provided you with a list of foods to avoid.

High fat foods that tend to decrease the processing of the food in the stomach. This can cause a build-up of acid. Listed below are ones to avoid:

- French fries
- Deep fried onion rings
- Potato chips
- Butter
- Whole milk
- Cheese
- Ice cream
- High fat sour cream
- High fat creamy salad dressings
- Creamy sauces and dips
- High fat cuts of red meat, such as marbled sirloin and prime rib

Spicy foods if they affect your GERD should be avoided, however, research has found that with regular exposure to capsaicin, which is the ingredient that makes chili peppers and powder spicy, can help you improve your GERD symptoms. But for this book, we are going to avoid spicy foods. Listed below is the spices you should avoid:

- Ground cinnamon
- Ground Mace
- Ground ginger
- Coriander
- Dill
- Parsley
- Garlic powder
- Fresh garlic
- Basil
- Thyme
- Tarragon
- Onion powder
- Dried onion pieces
- Black pepper
- Crushed red pepper flakes
- Tabasco sauce

- Chili powder
- Curry powder
- Cloves
- Mustard seed
- Nutmeg

Remember that all of your food choices should be monitored with a food journal so that you can be certain which foods affect your GERD. Not all of the spices will affect everyone, however, they will affect the majority of people.

Other foods you should avoid include dairy products. You should also avoid fatty foods, some fruits, some greasy foods, and vinegars. We have included a list below that has not been mentioned previously in the foods to avoid list.

- Chocolate
- Peppermint
- Spearmint

- Cider vinegar
- Rice vinegar
- Coffee
- Citrus juice
- Caffeinated or carbonated drinks
- Alcoholic beverages
- Beer
- Tea
- Coca-Cola
- Mint tea
- Whole milk or chocolate milk
- Doughnuts
- Croissants
- Tortilla chips
- Grapefruit juice
- Cranberry juice
- Peppers
- Radishes
- Beef
- Chicken nuggets Buffalo wings
- Macaroni with a rich sauce

- Milkshake
- Pickles
- Pastries
- Fry ups
- Curries
- Brownie
- Pasta prepared with creamy sauce or pesto
- Fried vegetables
- Fried meat
- Fried chicken
- Fried fish
- Sausage
- Pepperoni
- Bacon
- Hot dogs
- Ice cream
- High fat cakes, pies, and cookies

Why is it important to have a GERD meal plan?

Following a meal plan is a very important part of the treatment and maintenance of GERD. When we eat properly we can digest our food much more efficiently. Correcting our weight problems will eliminate our symptoms of GERD. Excess weight is one of the culprits to GERD. By being overweight we are blocking our ability to digest food, it is like putting a cinch on your stomach, applying pressure to the sphincter and relaxing the muscle due to stress and strain. The resulting factor would be GERD.

When we eat a GERD diet we are eating more healthy foods and allowing our bodies time to digest the food that we eat. This, in turn, allows our body to release the pressure on the esophageal sphincter and gives us a better chance at fighting the symptoms of GERD. Over time we can change our health by eating a healthier diet and we can start seeing results that will eliminate the GERD altogether.

Other things to consider:

• Smaller portion sizes allow for more control of your food intake and digestive abilities.
• Less acid-based foods prevent aggravating the stomach allowing the GERD to subside.
• More nutrient-rich foods allow you to stay full longer and need less food, which in turn allows you to lose weight.
• By decreasing the intake of sugar and

caffeine that you consume, you can eliminate the acid that results from consumption of these food items.

• Allow for more time to digest your food preventing GERD symptoms.

• When you get healthy, you decrease your needs for more medicines and in the long run lower your medical bills.

• Reduce inflammation in your stomach by eating all the right foods and keeping a food journal to know exactly what you can and can't eat.

• Prevent progressing your GERD to a more serious condition that is likely fatal.

• All of these allow for you to limit your medicine intake for GERD, which could potentially cause you more harm than good.

• By not being dependent on medicine you are not making your GERD worse nor are you adding the new and more dangerous diagnosis to your medical history.

Scheduling your strategy for your GERD Diet Meal Plan

When starting a new diet plan it is always best to have a strategy for the schedule you wish to use. In this section, we will discuss one aspect of scheduling strategy for your meal plan. There are several scheduling strategies that can be talked about in this section, but I would like to talk about your food diary journal. A food diary journal will help you know exactly what you can and cannot eat. This will help you plan your meal plan with only foods that are appropriate for your digestive system.

There are several steps you take to produce a workable food journal. Those are listed here.

• Start by picking out a nice book or journal that you will fill confident using daily.

• Make a chart for each day for the week leaving enough space to add in breakfast, lunch, dinner, snacks, and drinks. It should have separate spaces for the day of the week, the food you ate, the symptoms you experienced, and anything else you would like to notate.

• Start recording everything you eat. You should keep track of herbs, sauces, food items, and drinks.

• Then in the secondary space to the right record where or not you felt heartburn or GERD symptoms.

• Make sure you write down the accurate quantities that you ate.

• You will also need the day of time, the place you ate it at, like the restaurant

name. This can be added to one of the spaces for extra needed to know information.
- It is best to make a chart that is 4x4 squares. Per day.
- Record your food intake for a week or longer depending on what you find in your results.
- Use the food journal to build a meal plan out of for your GERD diet.

Sample meal plan for the GERD Diet Meal Plan

Here is a sample of how the GERD Diet Meal Plan will look when you start planning out yours.

Breakfast

- 1 cup of hot oatmeal
- 8-oz. of skim milk
- 0.50 cup of papaya slices

- 2 slices of whole wheat bread
- 1 tbsp. of peanut butter

Lunch

- Chickpea, tomato and Kale stew
- 2 slices Whole wheat bread
- An 8-oz glass of water
- 2 slices of avocado

Dinner

- Smoked salmon potato Tartine
- 8-oz water
- 1 cup of peaches with cream cheese
- 2 slices of whole wheat bread

Snacks

- Roasted Quince and cardamom popsicle- mid-morning
- Yoghurt parfait-mid-afternoon

Try this simple sample recipe for Breakfast.

Chia seeds can be soaked and as they soak they expand, this will help with the reduction of acid reflux.

Eat them in moderation because they do contain fat, however, they offer lots of fiber as well as protein.

Chia Breakfast Pudding

What's In It

- Skim milk (1 c.)
- Chia seeds (0.25 c.)
- Honey (2 Tbsp.)
- Alcohol-free Vanilla extract (0.50 tsp)
- Low-acid fruit, pears or nectarines (0.50 c.)

How It's Made

- Start by whisking the milk in a bowl with the other ingredients, minus the fruit.
- Whisk until completely blended.
- Cover the bowl and refrigerate the chia pudding overnight.
- The next day you can eat half of the pudding for breakfast and the other half for your mid-morning snack. Add some fruit to the pudding for extra nutrients and flavor.

CHAPTER SUMMARY:

3.1. In this chapter, we talked about why it is important to have a GERD diet meal plan and how to plan on out. We discussed what exactly to expect from a GERD diet meal plan and what not to include in your meals. We also discussed how the meal plan can help you reduce your acid reflux.

3.2. Next, we talked about building a scheduling strategy that will work and one part of the scheduling strategy that you can start with today.

3.3. The last part we gave you a simple sample breakfast recipe that will help you have a sample idea of what you can expect from the GERD Diet Meal Plan. We gave you the step by step instructions for making Chia Seed Pudding and explained why it is a great option for the GERD Diet Meal Plan.

YOUR QUICK START ACTION STEP:

Now that we have gone over everything you need to know about GERD and the GERD Diet Meal Plan, we are next going to give you recipes that will help you plan your GERD Diet Meal Plan without having to search for what is appropriate and find recipes that you can use. These are some of the best recipes online that can be used for the GERD Diet Meal Plan. I hope that you take some time out and scan through these recipes. I'm sure you will be pleased with the options that we have presented to you here.

Chapter 4: Breakfast

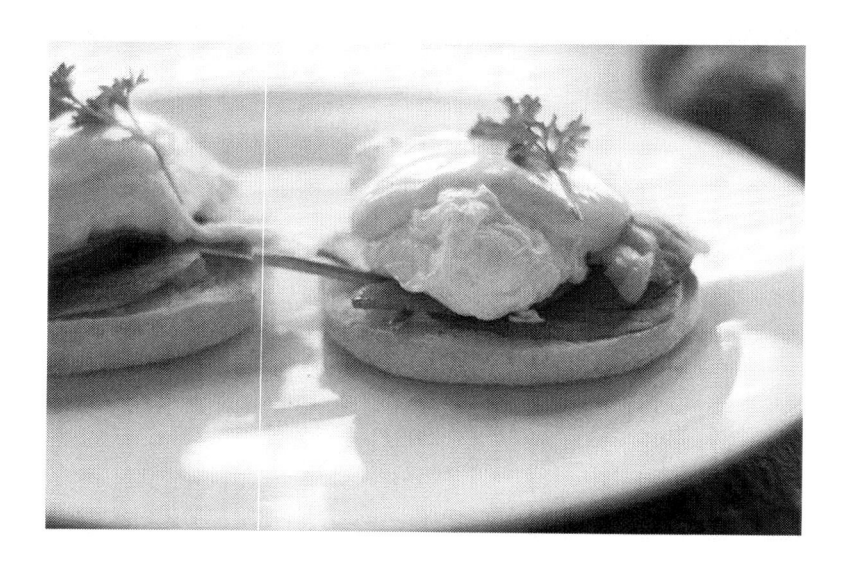

Chapter 4: Breakfast

This section of the book will provide you with breakfast recipes that can help you with preparing a GERD Diet Meal Plan. Now that we have covered everything about what GERD is and why you need a GERD diet Meal Plan. Up to this point, we have focused on the science. Now we will focus on the dietary needs. Food is not something to be afraid of. It is definitely not something we should overindulge in, however eating things that we like within a healthy range can benefit us in so many ways.

With GERD we have to be careful about what we eat so that we do not have symptoms. GERD can be very painful, and often times people just continue to eat the bad foods and take medications that Doctors are now finding create more health issues than they treat. This is not a healthy way of dealing with your GERD. SO in the next 7 chapters, we will help you have a well-balanced diet, get those foods that you love, and treat your GERD. Every recipe will have every detail we can provide to ensure that you are getting the exact information you need to continue your GERD health.

Coconut French Toast with Roasted Rhubarb and Hazelnut Orange Dukkha (Gluten and Dairy Free)

Serves 4

What's In It

- Roasted Rhubarb:
- Orange (1)
- Unrefined raw sugar (0.33 c.)

- Rhubarb (500 g)
- Hazelnut and orange Dukkha:
- Pinch of salt
- Cardamom (1 tsp)
- Ginger (0.25 tsp)
- Cinnamon (0.25 tsp)
- Fennel seeds (0.50 tsp)
- Coriander seeds (0.50 tsp)
- Shredded coconut (2 tbsp.)
- Sesame seeds (0.25 c.)
- Almonds (2 tbsp.)
- Hazelnut (0.25 c.)
- Gluten free bread (8 slices)
- Eggs (free range) (2 large)
- Coconut milk (0.50 c.)
- Almond milk (0.650 c.)
- Vanilla extract (1 tsp)
- Virgin coconut or olive oil

How it's Made

- Start with preheating your oven to 35 degrees f.
- Slice some rhubarb into pieces that are 2 cm long and place in a bowl. Scatter with sugar.
- Zest and grate some orange and set it aside to sue the Dukkha.
- Next juice orange and stir with rhubarb.
- Place the rhubarb on a baking sheet along with some juice and sugar that is left in the bowl.
- Roast 12 to 15 minutes, the rhubarb should be tender, not mushy. Remove it and set it to the side for later.
- When done with that, roast your hazelnuts and almonds on a baking sheet for 8 to 10 minutes, making sure to shake the pan so that they don't stick. Once they are done rub

the skin off of your hazelnuts and lay to the side to cool.

- Next toast your sesame seeds, coriander, coconut and fennel seeds in a dry frying pan that is heated to a temperature of medium to high heat. Once they are toasted, remove from heat and add to the food processor, mixing in the ground spices. Then the salt. Pulse the processor until they are finely ground up.
- Next, add the reserved orange zest.
- In a bowl whisk your eggs, coconut and almond milk and then the vanilla. Soak a few pieces of bread in the mix, allow it to sit in the mix for a bit. This helps it soak up enough mix.
- Heat your frying pan over the temperature of medium to high heat, then add in some oil. Place your French toast in the pan for a few

minutes per side. It should be golden when done.
- Serve them hot with rhubarb and Dukkha.
- Store left-overs in a fridge for 4 to 5 days.

Boysenberry, Lemon and Yoghurt Breakfast Pops

This recipe makes 8 servings

What's In It

- Gluten free muesli (0.50 c.)
- Lemon zest that is finely grated (1)
- Unsweetened Greek yoghurt (2 c.)
- NZ Boysenberries (1 c.)
- Honey (4 tbsp.)

How It's Made

- Start by adding in some boysenberries and honey into a small

boiler. The using your lid cover the boiler and cook on low until it is defrosted.
- Take off the lid and increase the heat slightly, along it to simmer for 2 minutes.
- Take it off the heat and crush your berries lightly, then set it aside.
- Mix the yoghurt with the remaining 3 tbsp. of honey and lemon zest, then mix it well.
- Now, divide your berries between the ice block molds and pour in the lemon yoghurt, the scoop a little granola on top.
- Press down the yoghurt to help it stick. Then insert your wooden stick in and freeze it for 4 hours or overnight.

- Run under some warm water to allow the pops to release from the mold.

Yogurt Parfait

This is a fresher alternative to the store-bought yogurt parfait and so much better.

What's In It

- Honey (2 Tbsp.)
- Plain non-fat yogurt (2 c.)
- Strawberries (.50 c.)

How It's Made

- Separate out your yogurt into two cups, for two individual servings.
- In each cup whisk 1 tbsp. of honey per cup to blend with the non-fat yogurt.

- Place in the refrigerator to chill overnight.
- In the morning take out one cup of yogurt and 0.50 c. of strawberries. Blend them together and enjoy for breakfast.
- A few hours later, for your mid-morning snack eat the other cup and another 0.50 c. of strawberries.
- Several GERD friendly fruits you can add would be melons, bananas, and peaches.

Avocado Toast

Although avocados are a high fat food, they are the exception to the high fat trigger for GERD. However, binging on them can still be not good.

What's In It

- Avocado (0.25 of one)

- Whole wheat toast (1 slice)

How It's Made

- Using a piece of whole wheat bread, that is toasted in the toaster, place 1 slice of avocado on the top.
- Eat the toast and enjoy.

Scrambled Eggs

Scrambled eggs are high in protein. They are a great low-volume breakfast food. Add in whole wheat toast with some butter or peanut butter spread and you have a complete meal.

What's In It

- Egg whites (2)
- Egg yolk (1)
- Whole Wheat toast

How It's Made

- By separating the egg whites form the yolk you can get the 2 egg whites and then save one of the yolks.
- Place in a frying pan on the stove over a temperature of medium to low heat to scramble the eggs.
- Place the toast in the toaster and toast one slice of it.
- Using butter or peanut butter spread a small bit on the toast.
- Place the eggs and the toast on a plate and enjoy.

Banana Smoothie

Whipping up a smoothie is a great way to get your breakfast on the go. Divide the smoothie into two separate servings and enjoy one for breakfast and one for a mid-morning snack.

What's In It

- Banana (1)
- Yogurt (0.50 c.)
- Almond butter (1 tbsp.)
- Skim Milk (1 c.)
- Honey (1 tbsp.)
- Crushed ice (1 c.)

How It's Made

- Start by placing your banana in the blender, along with the almond butter, yogurt, skim milk, and honey with the crushed ice.
- Blend it all together until smooth.
- Separate it to two separate cups.

Mango Pancakes

These are a great gluten free option for the GERD diet. This recipe makes 5 small pancakes, this makes 2 separate meals.

What's In It

- Water (2 c.)
- Coconut oil to grease the pan
- Almond nut butter (3 tbsp.)
- Oats (1.50 c.)
- Blueberries (1 c.)
- Mango (4 slices)
- Ripe bananas (2 ripe)

How it's made

- Start by preparing your fruit. First, you should peel your banana.
- Then, place your banana, mango, oats, water and almond butter into a food processor, blending it for a minute.
- Once blended, move it to a bowl and stir in the blueberries.
- Let it sit for a bit to allow the oats to soak up some of the liquid.

- Next, using a non-stick frying pan and a bit of the coconut oil for greasing, place the pan on the stove over a temperature of medium to low heat.
- Once the frying pan is heated properly, scoop a small portion of your mix into the pan.
- Let it cook for a bit allowing the edges to cook completely, and the center bubble.
- Flip the pancake over and let it continue to cook for about another 1 to 2 minutes.
- The top side should be browned and no longer runny.
- They should be small pancakes. You can enjoy two for breakfast and 2 for your mid-morning snack. Add some fruit on top for garnish.

Stewed Breakfast Apples

This meal can serve one person. It is a great way to get your fruit and feel like you are eating a healthy snack at the same time.

What's In It

- Granola
- Cinnamon (1 tsp)
- Coconut milk (0.50 can)
- Fresh ginger (0.50 of an inch)
- Raw honey (1 heap)
- Apples (2 red)
- Blueberries (1 handful)

How It's Made

- You want to start by peeling your apples. Then cut them into pieces that are bite-sized. Tossing the core out.

- Place some pieces in a boiler with some blueberries, some cinnamon, the honey, and then using coconut milk cover the bottom of the boiler.
- Let it cool on a low heat, simmering for a little bit.
- While cooking continues to add in liquid so that it does not stick.
- Next, peel your ginger and begin to grate it on to a plate
- Once you have the amount of ginger you need place it in the boiler with the other ingredients.
- Continue to cook for 20 minutes at this point the coconut milk should be all evaporated.
- Now, place your apples in a bowl and use your boiler to heat up the rest of your coconut milk for 2 minutes.
- Cover the apples with the coconut milk and add in your granola.

- Enjoy!

Coconut Cashew Chia Pudding

You should make this the day before you wish to eat it. Chia seeds add nutrients to any meal. It must sit for a few hours to thicken to a proper consistency.

What's In It

- Chia seeds (2 tbsp.)
- Lemon juice (2 tbsp.)
- Coconut milk (1 c.)
- Vanilla extract (1 tsp)
- Honey (2 tbsp.)
- Cashews (soaked for 3 hours) (1 c.)

How It's Made

- Start with mixing your cashews, coconut milk, honey, lemon juice, and vanilla extract in your blender. Blending until smooth.

- Move the finished ingredients to a glass container and blend in your chia seeds with a spoon.
- Place the mix into the refrigerator until the next day. This is when the pudding will thicken.
- Slice some strawberries into quarters.
- Separate the pudding into two cups.
- Starting by adding a layer of pudding and then adding in a layer of strawberries, then repeat.
- Eat one for breakfast and one for a mid-morning snack.

Easy Spinach Artichoke Quiche Cups

This recipe will provide you 12 individual cups. They are super easy to make and very enjoyable.

What's In It

- Spinach (drained) (1 package)
- Artichoke (hearts, drained and chopped) (1 14.5-oz. package)
- Eggs (5)

How it's Made

- Start by heating your oven to a temperature of 350-degrees f.
- Prepare you muffin pan by either lining them or using olive oil spray.
- Mix the spinach, artichoke, and eggs that have been whisked, together in a bowl.
- Scoop your mix into the muffin pans sections, equally.
- Place the pan in the oven and bake for 20 minutes.

- A toothpick should come out clean when inserted in the middle of a quiche.
- Eat 2 quiches for breakfast, and 2 for a min-morning snack. Freeze the rest for later.

Chapter 5: Soups

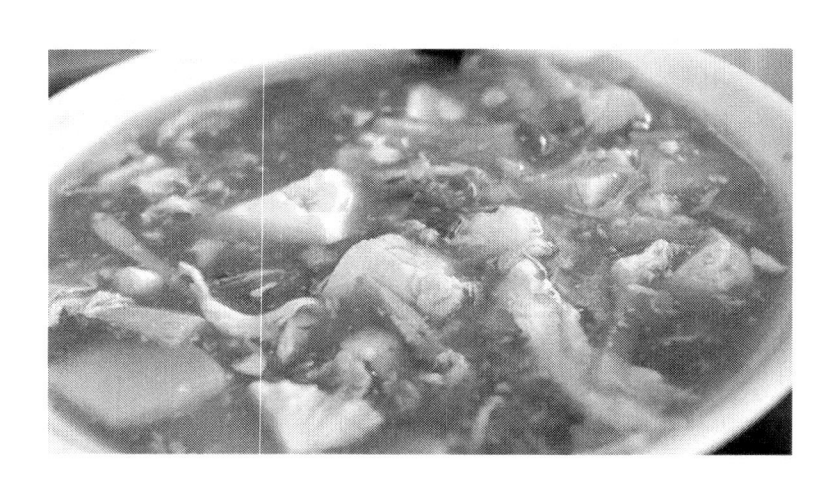

Chapter 5: Soups

Soups should be a staple meal option in any household. I have found that kids love soup. They don't realize they are eating all those yucky vegetables because soup is fun. The best thing about soup though is that it warms the stomach which prevents symptoms of GERD.

Chickpea, Tomato and Kale Stew with Herbed Yoghurt

This stew may have many ingredients, but it is delicious once you are done preparing it. It takes a matter of only minutes to prepare and its versatile, you could use kale or cabbage.

What's In It

- Ground turmeric (0.50 tsp)
- Fine sea salt (1 tsp)
- Raw sugar (0.50 tsp)
- Tomatoes (1 400-g)
- Tomato paste (2 tbsp.)
- Cold water (2 c.)
- Chickpeas (3 c.)
- Kale (0.50 bunch)
- Red wine vinegar or lemon juice (1 to 2 tsp)
- Smoked Paprika (0.50 tsp)
- Fennel seeds (0.50 tsp)
- Ground coriander (1 tsp)
- Cumin seeds (1 tsp)
- Bay leaf (1)
- Fresh thyme (3 sprigs)
- Garlic (2 cloves)
- Onion (1)
- Olive oil (2 tbsp.)

Coriander Yoghurt

- Lemon juice (0.50)
- Fine sea salt (0.50 tsp)
- Mint leaves (1 tbsp.)
- Coriander leaves (0.25 c.)
- Greek yoghurt (1 c.)

How It's Made

- Start by heating olive oil in a boiler add some onion and cook it for 5 minutes. Stirring until they are translucent.
- Next, add in some garlic thyme sprigs and cumin seeds, along with bay leaf.
- Stir well and continue to cook the ingredients for about a minute.
- Now, add in some spices, salts, and sugar and continue to cook for 30 seconds.

- Then, add in some tomatoes, tomato paste, water and chickpeas.
- Once you bring all of this to a boil you can reduce it and continue simmering while placing a lid on the boiler. Cook for a total of 10 minutes.
- Now, to make the yoghurt you should blend all the ingredients together int a bowl and stir until well blended.

Roasted Red Pepper and Sweet Potato Soup

What's in it

- Cream cheese (4.0-oz.)
- Lemon juice (1 tbsp.)
- Fresh cilantro (2 tbsp.)
- Sweet potato (3-4 c.)
- Vegetable broth (4 c.)

- Ground cumin (2 tsp)
- Ground coriander (1 tsp)
- Roasted red pepper (1 jar 12.0-oz.) (preserve liquid)
- Green chilis (1 can 4.0-oz.)
- Onions (2 medium)
- Olive oil (2 tbsp.)

How It's Made

- In a boiler or Dutch oven, start heating your olive oil over medium to high heat. Next, add in some onions and cook them until they are soft.
- Next add in some red peppers, cumin, green chilies, and coriander for flavor. Cook for 1 to 2 minutes.
- Using the reserved juice for the peppers, stir it together with the sweet potatoes and vegetable broth. Bring everything to a boil, then lower the heat and using a lid cover the pot.

Cook until your potatoes are tender. This should be about 10 to 15 minutes.
- Now, stir in cilantro and lemon juice.
- Let your soup cool off slightly.
- Next, put half of the soup into a blender with some cream cheese and process it until completely smooth. Add this back into the soup in the boiler and make sure it is heated through.
- Scoop into a bowl and serve.

Thai Pumpkin Soup

This is a simple 5 ingredient recipe that is sure to be a great option for the GERD diet Meal Plan. Although curry is sometimes inflammatory, this recipe is designed with GERD in mind. So, check your food journal and verify that you are not prone to GERD symptoms from the curry. If you are not prone to symptoms, then this meal will be one of your favorites.

What's In It

- Cilantro for garnish
- Coconut milk (1.75 c., holding back 1 tbsp.)
- Red chili pepper (1 large slice)
- Pumpkin puree (2 15.0-oz. cans)
- Chicken and vegetable broth (4 c.) (32.0-oz)
- Red curry paste (2 tbsp.)

How It's Made

- Place your boiler on the stove over medium heat and cook your curry paste. This should take about 1 minute. The paste should become fragrant.

- Next, add your chicken and vegetable broth and the pumpkin, stirring continuously.
- Cook the mix for about 3 minutes, at which time the soup should be bubbly.
- Next, add in the coconut milk and cook until the ingredients are hot. This should take about 3 minutes.
- Once the soup is done, ladle it into some bowls and garnish with a sprinkle of coconut milk and sliced red chilies. Garnish with cilantro leaves.

Ginger Ground Turkey Soup

Soup is great for meals on the go. You can get them ready the night before. Place them in a Thermos and be prepared for lunch the next day at work. This soup recipe makes 4 servings and is a great GERD Diet Meal Plan option. Ginger is soothing to the stomach and to your GERD while ground turkey is low in fat.

What's In It

- Chicken broth (4 c.)
- Carrot (2 slices) zucchini (chopped) (1)
- Peas (1 c.)
- Ginger root (grated, peeled) (1 tsp)
- Turkey breast (ground) (0.50 lbs.)

How It's Made

- Start by simmering your 4 c. of broth and ginger root along with the carrots and zucchini. Then place the peas in the broth and simmer all vegetables until they are soft.
- This should take 10 minutes.

- Next, in a skillet brown your turkey and add it to the soup.
- Simmer this for five minutes.
- Add seasonings that you like for flavor. Avoiding ones that trigger GERD.

Chapter 6: Salads

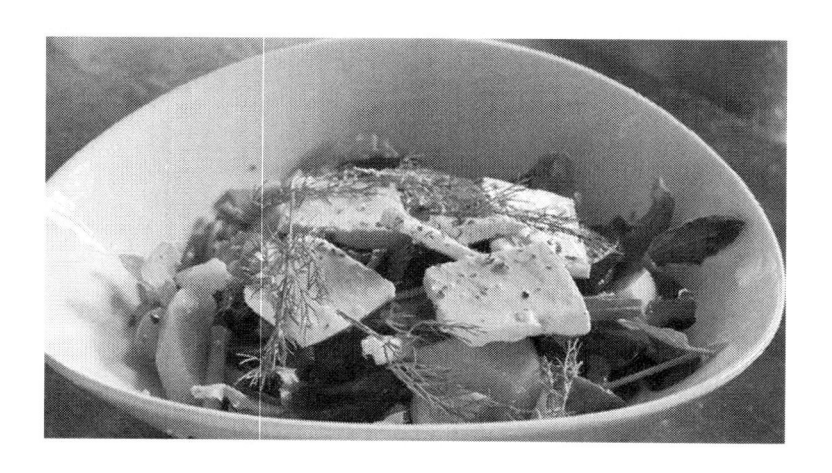

Chapter 6: Salads

Salads are everybody's favorite light lunch meal. The great thing about being on a diet is that anytime you go out to eat you are guaranteed that the restaurant will have a salad that you will love. In this section, we are all about salads. Although salads, in general, should be fine for GERD sufferers, some people will be affected by salad. So, tread lightly and keep a record in your food journal so you know what you can and can't have.

Winter Fruit Salad with Persimmons, Pears, Grapes, Pecans, and Agave-Pomegranate Vinaigrette

What's In It

- Pecans (cut lengthwise) (0.75 c.)

- Grapes (1 c.)
- Bosch Pears (1-inch cubes)
- Fuyu Persimmons (1-inch cubes)

Dressing

- Agave nectar (2 tbsp..)
- Peanut oil (1 tbsp..)
- Pomegranate flavored vinegar (1 tbsp..)
- Extra virgin olive oil (1 tbsp..)

How It's Made

- Start with whisking together all of your dressing ingredients so the flavors can mix for a while.
- Then, proceed to cut the fruit into chunks. Cut the grapes, persimmons, and pears. Place them in a bowl. Next, toss your fruit with some dressing.

- Place the salad in the fridge and let it chill.
- Once you are ready to serve the salad, add some pecan pieces.

Grilled Zucchini and spinach Salad with Roasted Capsicum (Red Pepper) Dressing

Serves 4 to 6

What's In It

Roasted Capsicum Dressing

- Fine Sea salt (to taste)
- Extra Virgin olive oil (0.50 c.)
- Red wine vinegar (3 tbsp.)
- Honey or brown rice syrup (vegan option) (0.50 tsp)
- Garlic (1 clove)
- Capsicum (red pepper) (1)

Ingredients

- Pine nuts (lightly toasted) (2 tbsp.)
- Baby spinach (1 bunch) (2 to 3 handfuls)
- Olive oil (shallow fry)
- Courgettis (4 medium)

How It's Made

- Start with setting your oven to a grill temperature.
- Next, place your capsicum halves on a baking sheet and little brush olive oil on the tops.
- Grill the capsicum for 8 to 10 minutes or until they are charred and black in spots.
- Take them from the oven and place into a bowl that is covered.
- Then, set them aside for 5 to 10 minutes.

- Now, peel off the skin and throw it out.
- Place grilled capsicum, honey, garlic and red wine vinegar into a blender and blend roughly.
- Next add in some olive oil in and continue to blend at high speed, they should be smooth and emulsified.
- Now slice your courgettis into 1 cm round pieces.
- Using a frying pan cook the courgetti, on medium to high heat, in batches, until they are golden brown on both sides. Continue cooking until they are all done and resting on a plate.
- To serve the courgettis arrange your spinach leaves and the grilled courgettis onto a platter and layer with some pine nuts and dressing.

Making sure that all the leaves are coated.
- You can store the left-over dressing in a glass jar and store in the fridge for 4 to 5 days.

Mediterranean Tuna Salad

This is an alternative to the traditional lettuce style salad. This salad could be served inside a lettuce wrap or a hollowed-out tomato if you do not get GERD symptoms from tomatoes.

What's In It

- Tomatoes (if you like) (2 large)
- Lemon juice (1 tbsp.)
- Fresh basil (2 tbsp. chopped)
- Capers (1 tbsp.)
- Fire roasted red peppers (2 tbsp.)
- Kalamata or mixed olives (0.25 c.)
- Red onions (minced) (2 tbsp.)

- Mayonnaise (0.25 c.)
- Tuna (2 5.0-oz cans)

How It's Made

- Start by adding in all the ingredients, minus the tomatoes, into a large bowl. Stir them to combine all the ingredients together. Slice tomatoes into $1/6^{th}$, but do not cut all the way.
- Slowly pry it open and begin to scoop the tuna salad into the middle.
- Can serve in a pita pocket, on a bed of lettuce, some crackers, and a sandwich.

Lunch Salad

This salad is a great GERD diet option and can be a very satisfying meal. It is filled with so many good nutrients and vegetables that you will be satisfied.

What's in It

- kale, spinach, lettuce each (0.50 c.)
- Veggies such as peas, broccoli, carrots, or zucchini (0.50 c.)
- For meat, one of these will do. Deli turkey, chicken breast, fish, shellfish like halibut or shrimp (3.0-oz.)

Dressing

- low fat buttermilk (0.50 c.)
- plain, non-fat yogurt (0.50 c.)
- honey (1 tsp)
- Dijon mustard (1 tbsp.)
- Fresh dill (1 tbsp.) (chopped)

How It's Made

- Start with chopping your salad mix so that it is bite size pieces.
- In a separate bowl mix your dressing ingredients with a whisk.

- Place your salad mix into a bowl and use 3 tbsp. of dressing on top of your salad.
- Place the left overs in the fridge sealed tightly for up to a week.

Chapter 7: Snacks

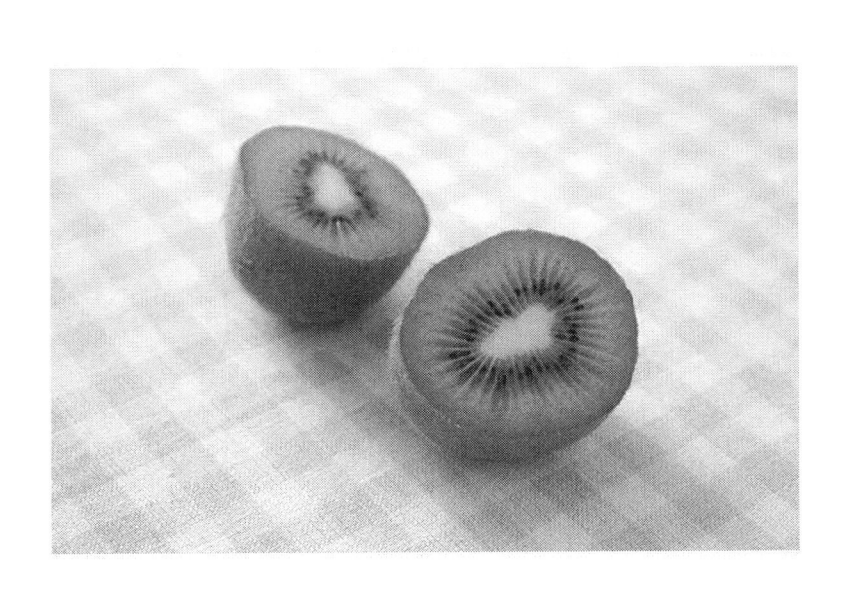

Chapter 7: Snacks

Roasted Carrot Hummus

Adding carrots to hummus brings a lovely sweetness to this dip.

Serves 4 to 6

What's In It

- Selection of baby vegetables, and cracker
- Warm water (2 to 4 tbsp.)
- Lemon juice (2 tbsp.)
- Tahini (2 tbsp.)
- garlic (2 cloves)
- chickpeas (1.50 c.)
- fine sea salt and pepper
- olive oil
- cumin seeds (0.50 tsp)
- carrots (2 large)

How It's Made

- Start with heating the oven to a temperature of 400 degrees f.
- Slice some carrots and transfer them to a baking dish.
- Toss you cumin seeds, and olive oil with seal salt all over the baking dish.
- Mix it well and then roast 25 to 30 minutes, turning it once or twice during the cooking process. Cook until they are tender and just starting to have color. Take them off of the heat and set them to the side to cool.
- Next, drain some chickpeas and rinse well. Place some garlic into the food processor and finely chop, adding in the chickpeas, some roasted carrot, lemon juice, and tahini, warm water about 2 tbsp..
- Blend it all together while adding water as needed. The hummus should be smooth.

- Place in a ramekin and add crudité for dipping.

Lemon Posset a La Poires Au Chocolat

What's in It

- Lemon juice (2 tbsp.)
- Caster sugar (50 g)
- Cream (150 ml)

How It's Made

- Start by pouring your cream into a boiler.
- Then, pour in your sugar.
- Heat the sugar over medium heat to dissolve it.
- Turn your heat up to high, when you see bubbles, cook it for 3 more minutes.

- The mix should vigorously bubble while cooking.
- When the timer goes off, take the pan off of the heat and clock one more minute.
- When it dings again stir in some lemon juice.
- Let it sit for 15 minutes then separate between two ramekins.
- Cover the ramekins with cling film and place in the fridge to chill.
- Let it sit for an hour.

Brazil Nut, Cacao and orange Granola

This makes about 8 servings

What's In It

- Cacao nibs (50 g)
- Honey (4 tbsp.)
- Zest and juice of an orange (1.50)

- Rape seed oil or olive oil (50 ml)
- Salt (pinch)
- Pumpkin seeds or sunflower seeds, or blend (150 g)
- Whole brazil nuts (1 c.)
- Porridge oats (350 g)

How It's Made

- Start by heating the oven to a degree of 350 f. using parchment paper line a couple of baking sheets.
- Place your oats, nuts salt, and seeds in a bowl. Mix everything together and pour your oil in mixing it together. Evenly distributing the ingredients.
- Mix the orange zest, orange juice, and honey and then pour the oats in and mix it all together. Using your hands will help in this case.

- Spread your mix out in the trays ad place in the oven. Bake for 45 to 50 minutes, once golden brown, give the mix a stir half way through the cooking process.
- Place the granola on the counter and cool it allowing it to crisp up. Stir in your cacao nibs and place all of it in an airtight container. Serve as snack or breakfast with some vanilla yoghurt.

Almost Raw Kiwi Fruit and Ginger Cheesecake

Due to the maple syrup, this recipe is not completely raw. Alternatively, you can use honey, but a smaller amount since it is sweeter. You can also add a bit of spinach to the green layers to get a brighter color. This does not change the flavor.

What's In It

- Virgin coconut oil (1 tbsp.)
- Whole raw almonds (0.666 c.)
- Dried Dates roughly chopped (1.50 c.)

Filling:

- Raw cashew nuts (soaked overnight in cold water) (3 c.)
- Virgin coconut oil (0.75 c. and 1 tbsp.)
- Lemon and lime juice 0.50 c.)
- Maple syrup or your favorite liquid sweetener (0.50 c.)
- Vanilla extract (1 tsp)
- Fine sea salt (0.25 tsp)
- Ginger (finely grated) (3 tbsp.)
- Spinach leaves (small handful) (optional)
- Green kiwi fruit (3 peeled)

- Gold kiwi fruit (1 peeled)

How It's Made

- Start with making the base, by lining a 28x18cm pan with some baking paper, making sure the paper overlaps the pan. Place the dates, coconut oil, and almonds into the food processor. Then blend on high until chopped fine.
- Now, press the mixture into the tin, use the spoon to pack down the nuts firmly.
- Next, make the filling by placing the cashews, after drained with the coconut oil, maple syrup, lemon juice, vanilla, and salt all into a blender.
- Now, blend on high until smooth. Transfer half the mix to a bowl and

add the ginger to the mix remaining in the blender.
- Continue to blend on high until smooth.
- Pour the ginger over the base and place it into the freezer, allowing it to cool.
- Now, get your spinach and 2 green kiwi fruits plus the reserved filling and add some coconut oil in the blender, do not rinse the blender first. Start to blend on high until smooth.
- Remove the mix from the freezer and pour kiwi filling over the bottom layer.
- Using a spoon smooth it out and place in the refrigerator for 4 to 5 hours, or overnight, until it is firmly set.

- Now, slice your green and gold kiwi into thin slices and lay the on top of the cheese cake.
- Slice the cake and serve. What is left over store it in the fridge covered for 5 to 7 days or freezer up to a month.

Orange jelly with Golden Kiwi Fruit and Granita (gluten free and vegan)

This recipe takes 4 to 6 hours to set and is a great snack for mid-morning snack time. To find the agar powder you should check an Asian grocer or a health food store. Agar is a vegan gelatin alternative made from seaweed. You must boil it to activate its setting properties and it must then be set at room temperature. Green kiwi is to sour so golden kiwi is best used for this recipe.

What's In It

- Agar powder (1 tsp)
- Palm sugar or unrefined raw sugar (2 tbsp.)
- Squeezed Orange juice (500 ml 2.0 c.)

Golden Kiwi fruit granita

- Lemon juice and lime (1 tsp)
- Golden kiwi fruit (200 g)
- Cold water (0.25 c.)
- Grated palm sugar or unrefined raw sugar (2 tbsp.)

How It's Made

- Start with adding in your orange juice, agar powder, and grated palm sugar in a boiler and set it over medium to high heat, bringing it to a boil. Continue to stir often to keep

the agar powder from settling at the bottom.
- Boil all of this for 1 minute.
- Now, take it off of the heat and set it to the side for a second.
- Grab some glasses, 4 will do. And scoop the orange juice evenly into each glass, set them aside in the fridge and cool allowing them to set.
- Chill them overnight in the refrigerator.
- Now, make your granita by combining palm sugar and water in a boiler. Continue to stir while dissolving the sugar.
- Boil the ingredients for 10 seconds and then remove it from the heat, set it to the side, allowing it to cool until it is nearly cold.
- Now, place the kiwi fruit, syrup, and lime juice into the processor and

- blend it until smooth, keeping the little black seeds still intact.
- Move the mix to a shallow dish that is freeze proof and move it to the freezer for 6 hours or for one night.
- The next day, take the jellies and granita out of the fridge and use a fork to scrape the granite mix to form some small ice crystals. Move it to a container and freeze for a little bit, making sure it doesn't melt while you are making ice shavings.
- Serve the granita piled high on the orange jellies and eat them right away.

Rhubarb, Apple and Ginger Muffin Recipe (Gluten and Dairy Free)

What's In It

- Ginger (0.50 tsp)

- Gluten free baking powder (2 tsp)
- Brown rice flour (0.25 c. fine)
- Cinnamon (0.50 tsp)
- Organic cornflower or true arrowroot (2 tbsp.)
- Buckwheat flour (0.50 c.)
- Linseed meal (1 tbsp.)
- Crystallized ginger (finely chopped) (2 tbsp.)
- Raw sugar (0.25 c.)
- Almond meal (ground almonds) (0.50 c.)
- Vanilla extract (1 tsp)
- Free-range egg (1 large)
- Olive oil (0.25 c.)
- Rice or almond milk (0.33 c and 1 tbsp.)
- Apple (peeled, cored, finely diced) (1 small)
- Rhubarb (1 c.)

How It's Made

- Start by heating the oven to a temperature of 350 degrees f. Grease the muffin tin or place paper cups in them.
- Place some almond meal, ginger, sugar, and linseed meal into a bowl. Then using a sieve place your flour and baking powder plus spices. Whisk to blend them evenly. Stir your rhubarb and apple into the flour mixture. In another bowl start to mix your milk, eggs, oil, and vanilla extract whisking to make sure it is all blended together.
- Next, pour the liquid mix into the dry mix, and stir to blend it all together.
- Now, evenly scoop the mix into cups in muffin tin, and place them in the oven for 20 to 25 minutes, at which

time the muffins should rise. They will be golden brown around the edges.
- Once done remove the muffins form the oven and set aside to chill at room temperature for 5 minutes. Transfer them to a wire cooling rack and let them continue to cool.
- You can serve them warm or cooled.
- They are best if eaten the day of but can be eaten the next day and up to 3 days if stored in air tight container or frozen in the freezer.

Chapter 8: Lunch

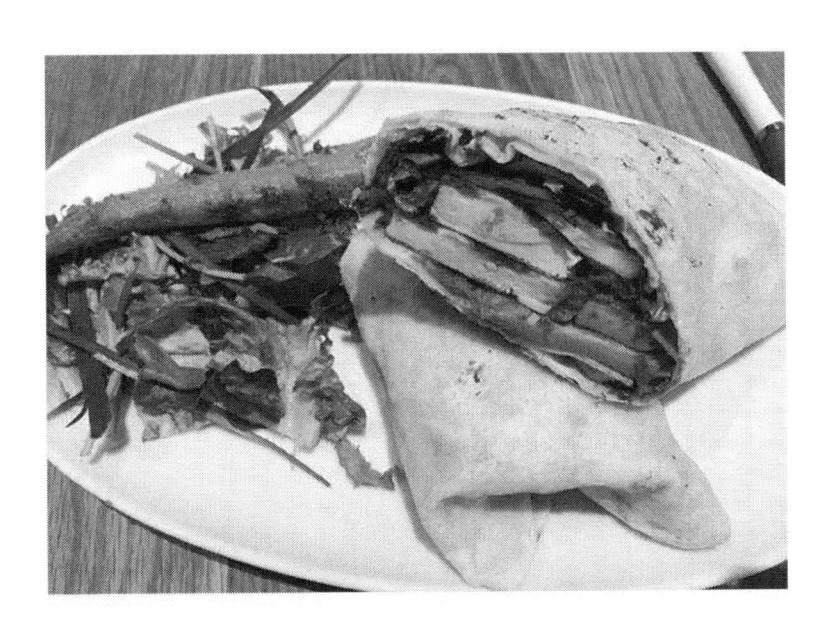

Chapter 8: Lunch

Orange Roasted Asparagus with Halloumi and Mint

Serves 4

What's In It

- Mint (handful)
- Olive oil
- Halloumi (200 g)
- Fine sea salt and pepper
- Honey (1 tsp)
- Lemon juice (1 tbsp.)
- Extra virgin olive oil (2 tbsp.)
- Orange juice (3 tbsp.)
- Zest of a small orange (1)
- Asparagus (2 bunches)

How It's Made

- Start by heating your oven to a temperature of 200 degrees. Trim

your asparagus and place it into a baking sheet. Add your orange zest, olive oil, juice, lemon juice, salt, pepper, and honey in a bowl. Pour your sauce mix over the asparagus place them in the oven and roast for 15 to 20 minutes. They should be tender when done.
- When they are almost cooked, heat up your frying pan over a temperature of medium to high and add in a splash of olive oil and cook your halloumi for 1 minutes
- The halloumi should take about 1 minute and be golden.
- When serving plate, the asparagus and some orange dressing on the plate, top it with the halloumi and mint leaves.
- Serve warm.

Green Tomato and Ginger Chutney

It is recommended to use a Muscovado Sugar, but it is not necessary.

Makes 6 to 8 medium jars

What's In It

- Dried chili flakes
- Cumin seeds (1 tbsp.)
- Ginger (2 tbsp.)
- Cider vinegar (2 c.)
- Sugar (500 g)
- Fine sea salt (4 tsp)
- Raisins or sultanas (250 g)
- Onion (500 g)
- Apples (500 g)
- Green tomatoes (2 kg)

How It's Made

- Start by adding all the ingredients in the boiler and bring it to a rolling boil.
- Stir the ingredients as it dissolves the sugar.
- Once the sugar is dissolved reduce your heat and let it gently simmer, cooking for a while longer.
- The sauce should be thick, this takes 1 hour.
- Next, pour it into hot sterilized jars, using the lid seal the jar.
- Chutney should be stored in a cool dark place for up to 12 months.
- Once you open it, place in the fridge.
- Using whole wheat toast smear onto bread or use crackers for a treat.

Turkey and Quinoa Stuffed Bell Pepper

What's In It

- Quinoa (1 c.)
- Chicken broth (1 c.)
- Tomato sauce (1 c.)
- Garlic (2 tsp)
- Spinach (1 c.)
- Sweet onion (0.25 c.)
- Mushrooms (1 c.)
- Ground Turkey (1.25 lbs.)
- Yellow peppers (3 large)

How It's Made

- In a boiler prepare you quinoa and cook it per the instructions on the box.
- During this time sauté the vegetables in your frying pan with some olive oil.
- In 5 minutes add in your ground turkey and some garlic and vegetables.

- Continue to cook over medium heat, cooking till the turkey is almost done.
- Next, add your tomato sauce and half your chicken broth. Simmering until your turkey is cooked all the way. Some of the excess liquid should be cooked off.
- Heat your oven to a temperature of 400 degrees f.
- While your turkey is simmering, prepare your bell peppers by washing them and then cutting them in half. Next, remove the seeds, as well as, stems.
- Now, spray the pan with some olive oil and lay your bell peppers in the pan.
- When your quinoa is cooking, place it into the pan, with some turkey and vegetables. Stir it all together and

then stuff your bell pepper with the mix. The bell peppers should be full.
- Pour your chicken broth into the pan.
- Cover with some foil and bake for a total of 30 to 35 minutes at a temperature of 400 degrees f.
- Serve and enjoy!

Honey and Orange Roasted Carrots with Whipped Feta and Pickled Radish

This should be prepared a day in advance, even further in advance if you want the radish pickles to turn fluorescent pink.

Serves 4 to 6

What's In It

Pickled Radishes

- Fine sea salt (0.50 tsp)
- Raw sugar (4 tsp)
- Apple cider vinegar (0.25 c.)
- Radish (2 bunches, approx. 12 to 14)

Ingredients

- Flat leaf parsley and mint leaves
- Medjool dates (2 fresh)
- Fine sea salt and black pepper
- Orange zest and juice
- Cumin seeds (0.50 tsp)
- Honey (1 tbsp.)
- Olive oil (3 tbsp.)
- Baby Carrots (500 g)

Whipped Feta

- Plain yoghurt (0.25 c.)
- Soft feta (200 g)

How It's Made

- Start with making the pickled radish by slicing the radishes into some thin rounds, using a mandolin.
- Combine your radishes with your apple cider vinegar, salt, and raw sugar. Set this aside for 2 to 4 hours, or overnight. Stirring occasionally.
- Next heat your oven to a temperature of a375 degrees f.
- While the oven is heating trim the tops off of the carrots, leave 2 cm.
- Lay them in a single layer on a baking sheet.
- Mix your olive oil, cumin seeds, zest and juice or orange, and honey in a bowl. Continue whisking to blend.
- Season with salt and pepper and then pour the ingredients over the carrots.

- Roast the mix for 30 to 35 minutes, continue to stir, making sure the meal is tender and golden.
- Once done take it out of the oven and set to the side to cool while you blend the feta and yoghurt in your processor.
- To serve the meal, scoop some feta onto each plate, and then top it with roasted carrots, drain your radish pickles and toss them on top using a few slices of medjool dates. Garnish with parsley and mint.

Spicy Sweet Potato Black Bean Burgers with Avocado-Cilantro Crèma Sprouts

What's In It

- For the Avocado-Cilantro Crèma: Non-GERD ingredient suggestions: Hot Sauce, Salt
- Lime juice (1tsp)
- Chopped cilantro (2 tbsp.)
- Low-fat sour cream or plain Greek yogurt (0.25 c.)
- Ripe avocado (0.50 large)
- For burgers: whole grain hamburger buns (gluten free) (6)
- Olive oil or coconut oil
- Gluten free oat flour (0.25)
- Spicy Cajun seasoning (2 tsp)
- Cumin (1 tsp)
- Jalapeno (0.50)
- Cilantro (0.50 c.)
- Garlic (2 cloves)
- Red onion (0.50 c.)
- Sweet potato (1 large)
- Black beans (1 can)

- Quinoa (0.50 c.)

How It's Made

- Start by rinsing the quinoa with cold water in a mesh strainer, then place it in a medium boiler and bring 1 cup of water to a boil, adding in the quinoa after it begins to boil. Once quinoa is boiling reduce the heat and using a lid cover the boiler.
- It should take 15 minutes for it to simmer at which time the quinoa will absorb the water. Remove the boiler from the heat and place it to the side so it can cool for 10 minutes. This should produce about 1.50 cups of quinoa.
- Now, using a fork, poke your sweet potato several times, then place the potato in the microwave for 3 to 4 minutes. The sweet potato should be

soft and cooked all the way through. Make sure not to overcook the sweet potato, since it will be to hard.
- When the potato is done cooking and cooled remove the skin.
- Next place the beans, garlic, sweet potato, red onion, cilantro, cumin, Cajun seasoning, in the food processor bowl and transfer the mix to a bowl and a mix with quinoa.
- Next, mix in your oat and bran flour, but just enough to shape the patties.
- Divide into 6 patties that are equal size, then place on parchment paper. Place in refrigerator for 30 minutes, this helps he patties bind together.
- To make the avocado-cilantro crèma in you need to combine in a food processor some sour cream, diced avocado, lime juice, and cilantro. Continue to blend until smooth.

Place into fridge until they are ready to serve.
- To cook burgers, you need to heat your frying pan over a temperature of medium to high heat. Spray the frying pan with some olive oil spray and fry the burger until they are golden brown on both sides. This takes 3 to 4 minutes per side. Serve the burgers with Crèma, sprouts, and top with your desired toppings.

Kale Caesar Salad with Grilled Chicken Wrap

What's In It

- Lavash Flat bread (2)
- Olive oil (0.125 c.)
- Lemon juice (0.125 c.)
- Honey (1 tsp)
- Garlic, (1 clove)

- Dijon mustard (0.50 tsp)
- Cherry Tomatoes (1 c.)
- Coddled Egg (0.50)
- Curly Kale (6 c.)
- Grilled chicken (thinly sliced) (8.0-oz.)
- Parmesan cheese (shredded) (0.25 c.)

How It's Made

- In a bowl place your coddled egg, mustard, garlic, honey, and lemon juice along with the olive oil.
- Whisk all the ingredients to form the dressing. Season for flavor.
- Next, add some kale, chicken, and cherry tomatoes. Toss the ingredients to coat with dressing and 0.25 c. of parmesan.

- Spread out your flatbreads and evenly layer the salad on top of the wraps. Now, sprinkle each with 0.25 c. of parmesan
- Now, roll up the wraps and slice in half.
- Eat one half for lunch and save the other side for later.

Sweet Potato with Cottage Cheese

Cottage cheese is an excellent source of low fat protein. It is also great for potato toppings

What's In It

- Sweet potato (1 potato or 0.50 cup)
- Cottage cheese (0.50 c.)
- Carrots (4 baby)

How It's Made

- Start with poking holes into the sweet potato and place it in the microwave for about 6 minutes. It should be soft when done.
- Next, top it with cottage cheese and serve with the baby carrots on the side.
- If the potato is more than 0.50 of a cup, then divide it and place in the fridge till later for the mid-evening snack.

Turkey and Cream Cheese Wrap

Cream cheese that is nonfat is a great fat-free option for any wrap. Spreading cream cheese on a whole wheat tortilla is a wonderful way to add flavor and no calories.

What's in It

- A whole wheat tortilla

- Nonfat cream cheese (1 tbsp.)
- Dijon mustard (2 tsp)
- Deli turkey slices (3.0-oz.)
- Alfalfa sprouts (0.25 c.)

How it's Made

- Start by wiping the nonfat cream cheese on the whole wheat wrap.
- Next smear some Dijon mustard onto the wrap.
- Now, place your deli slices on the wrap and a cup of alfalfa sprouts.
- Wrap the wrap and cut it in half.

Place half on your plate and the other half in the fridge for later.

Chapter 9: Dinner

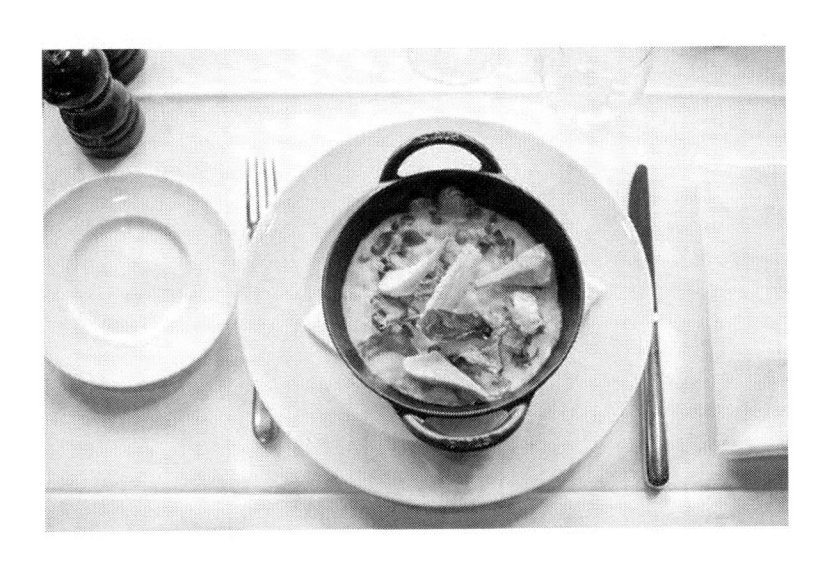

Chapter 9: Dinner

Roasted Eggplant with Pomegranate Molasses Dressing

Pomegranate Molasses can be found at supermarkets of health food stores. If you are vegan use brown rice syrup instead of the honey.

Servers 4 to 6

What's In It

Pomegranate Dressing

- Extra virgin olive oil (4 tbsp.)
- Pomegranate molasses (2 tbsp.)
- Lemon juice (3 tbsp.)
- Honey (1 tbsp.)

Ingredients

- Fresh mint leaves
- Pomegranate seeds (0.50)

- Ground black pepper and sea salt (for flavor)
- Olive oil (3 tbsp.)
- Eggplants (2 medium)

How It's Made

- Heat the oven to a temperature of 400 degrees f.
- Now using a brush, coat two baking sheets with some olive oil and then lay your eggplant slices in a single layer across the sheet.
- Brush the tops with the oil and season it. Roast the eggplant with 15 to 20 minutes until golden on the bottom.
- Flip each one of the eggplants and cook for 10 more minutes. They should be golden on both sides and tender. Remove from the oven and

set it to the side and cool to room temperature.
- Now, add in honey and pomegranate molasses together in a bowl.
- Now, add you lemon juice and olive oil, then whisk.
- Serve by transferring eggplant rounds to a platter and using your dressing, drizzle and scatter with pomegranate seeds and mint leaves.
- Store your left-over dressing in a jar for up to 1-week in the fridge.
- Serve and enjoy!

One Pan Lemon Herb Salmon and Zucchini

What's In It

- Olive oil (2 tbsp.)
- Zucchini (chopped) (4)

Salmon

- Fresh parsley leaves (2 tbsp.)
- Salmon fillets (4 5.0-oz.)
- Dried thyme (0.25 tsp)
- Dried rosemary (0.25 tsp)
- Garlic (2 cloves)
- Dried oregano (0.50 tsp)
- Dijon mustard (1 tbsp.)
- Lemon juice (2 tbsp.)
- Brown sugar (2 tbsp.)

How It's Made

- Start by heating your oven to a temperature of 400 degrees f. Using olive oil spray coat the baking sheet.
- Then get a bowl out and whisk in the brown sugar, Dijon mustard, garlic, dill, oregano, lemon juice, rosemary, and thyme. Season to taste. Now, lay it aside.

- Put your zucchini flat on the baking sheet and drizzle with olive oil. Next, add In some Salmon on the zucchini brushing with the herb mix.
- Place the baking sheet in the oven and cook the fish sis flaky when touched with a fork. This should take about 16 to 18 minutes.
- Serve while hot and use parsley to garnish.

Smoked Salmon Potato Tartine

What's in it

Potato Tartine

- Clarified Butter (2 tbsp.)
- Russet Potato (1 large)

Toppings

- Minced chives (garnish)
- Hardboiled egg (0.50)

- Red onions (2 tbsp.)
- Capers (2 tbsp.)
- Garlic (0.50 clove)
- Lemon (zest of a half)
- Smoked Salmon (thinly sliced)
- Minced chives (1.50 tbsp.)
- Soft goat cheese (4.0-oz.)

How It's Made

- Assemble the toppings by mixing the goat cheese, lemon zest, and garlic in a bowl. Gently stir it all together. Add in some chives for garnish.
- Then use seasoning to flavor the chopped onion and hardboiled egg.
- Now, mix your potato tartine by working quickly and grate the potato into a bowl using large grater holes. Using a paper towel squeeze the potato strings.

- Start by heating clarified butter in an 8 to 10-inch frying pan over the temperature of medium to high heat. Once the pan is hot, place the grated potato and shape it roughly into a large circle.
- Using the back of the spoon, press the mix to compact it. Cook it gently for 8 to 10 minutes until the bottom is golden brown.
- Using a spatula and flip the potato cake to the other side and continue to cook for 8 to 10 minutes or until golden brown and crispy.
- Remove them from the pan and place them on a cooling rack, allowing them to cool until they are luck warm or room temperature.
- Assemble the tartine with a potato cake and goat cheese spread on top. Next layer your smoked salmon with

some red onion, some hard-boiled eggs, and capers (if you like)
- Now, garnish with fresh chives.
- Cut the wedges and serve.

Italian-Styled Stuffed Red Peppers

What's In It

- Low calorie sweetener (1 packet)
- Chopped spinach (0.50 c.)
- Parmesan cheese (if it does not bother your GERD) (2 Tbsp.)
- Garlic powder (1 tsp)
- Basil/oregano (1 tsp)
- Spaghetti sauce (2 c.) (if it doesn't bother your GERD)
- Red bell peppers (3)
- Lean ground Turkey (1 lbs.)

How It's Made

- Start by heating the oven to 450 degrees f. using some parchment paper, line your baking sheet. Using olive oil spray coat the parchment paper.
- Next, wash your red peppers, and cut the stems off.
- Now, remove the stems and the centers.
- Slice your peppers into separate lengthwise halves. Removing the seeds and insides, make sure it is all cleaned out.
- Set the peppers on the baking sheet and prepare the rest of the ingredients.
- Cook your ground turkey in a pan over medium to high temperature. Stir to break up the turkey, when cooked through add in your sauce and some seasoning. Stir to continue

cooking while adding the spinach. Continue cooking till everything is blended.
- Scoop 0.50 c. of turkey mix into your peppers.
- Layer with some parmesan cheese over the peppers.
- Place the pan in the oven and cook for 20 to 30 minutes until the cheese melts and is lightly golden.
- Remove from the oven, set it to the side and let it cool.
- Enjoy!

Baked Tilapia with Pecan Rosemary Topping

What's In It

- Tilapia fillets (4 4.0-oz each)
- Coconut palm sugar or brown sugar (0.50 tsp)

- Cayenne pepper (1 pinch)
- Egg white (1)
- Olive oil (1.50 tsp)
- Fresh rosemary (chopped) (2 tsp)
- Whole wheat panko breadcrumbs (0.33 c.)
- Raw pecans (0.33 c.)

How It's Made

- Start by heating your oven to 350-degrees f.
- Next, in a small baking pan, mix together your pecans, breadcrumbs, coconut palm sugar, cayenne, rosemary, and olive oil. Toss it all to coat with the mix.
- Bake the ingredients until the pecan mix is light golden brown
- This should only take 7 to 8 minutes.

- Increase your heat to 400 degrees and coat your baking dish with some olive oil spray.
- Next, in your baking dish, whisk you egg whites together, and using one tilapia at a time, dip the fish into an egg and then the pecan mix. Lightly coat the fish, making sure both sides of the fish are coated. Place the fillet in your dish.
- Bake the tilapia until it is cooked all the way through, this should be about 10 minutes.

Curried Potatoes with Poached Eggs

This recipe only takes a few ingredients and is full of flavor. This is a perfect lunch recipe or dinner.

What's In It

- Cilantro (0.50 bunch)
- Eggs (4 large)
- Tomato Sauce (15.0-oz. can)
- Olive oil (1 tbsp.)
- Curry powder (2 tbsp.)
- Russet potatoes (2) (2 lbs.)
- Ginger (1-inch)
- Garlic (2 coves)

How It's Made

- Start with washing your potatoes and then cut them into 0.75-inch cubes. Place your potatoes in a boiler and cover the potatoes with water. Cover the boiler using the lid and bring it all to a boil over a temperature of high heat. Boil your potatoes for 5 to 6 minutes. They should be tender. Using a fork pierce the potatoes with

a fork to check that they are done. Drain the potatoes in a strainer.
- During the boiling of the potatoes start your sauce.
- Now peel your ginger and scrape your skins off into a bowl. Then grate your ginger in a cheese grater. Then proceed to mince your garlic.
- Now, add the ginger, garlic, and olive oil to a large deep-frying pan. Sauté your ginger with your garlic over a medium temperature. This should only take 1 to 2 minutes. They should then be soft and fragrant.
- Next, add in your curry powder and sauté for another minute, this is toasting the spices.
- Then, pour your tomato sauce into the frying pan. Stir all the ingredients to mix it together. Turn your heat up to a temperature of

medium heat and make sure the sauce is cooked all the way through. Taste your sauce to make sure it is good.
- Now add in the cooked potatoes with all the other ingredients and stir to coat everything. Add water if the sauce is to dry or paste.
- Make small wells in the potatoes, you will need 4. Then crack an egg and place it in each well. Using a lid, place it on the frying pan and let it simmer. The eggs should be simmering in the sauce for 6 to 10 minutes, they will be cooked all the way through.
- Right before serving chop cilantro and use it for garnish.

Chapter 10: Desserts

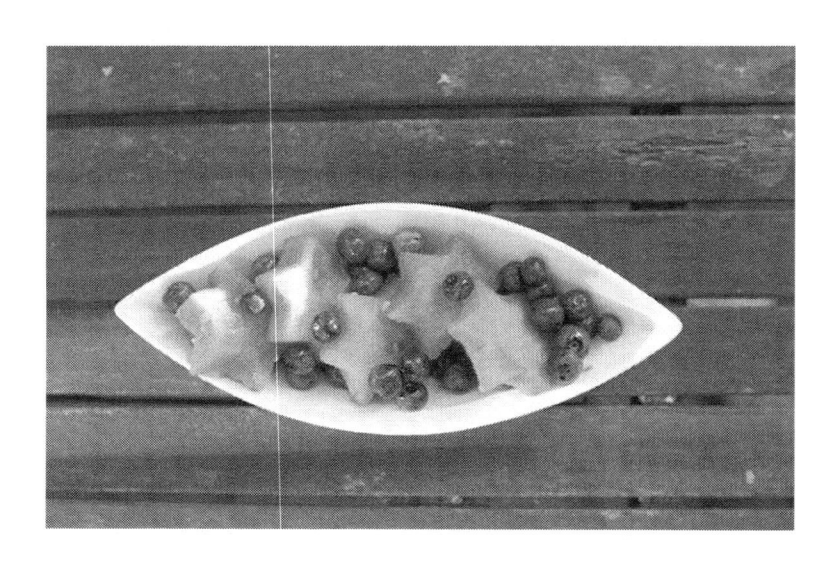

Chapter 10: Desserts

Gluten Free Blueberry, Lemon, Coconut Cake

This is a simple butter cake that can be topped with some of the best fruits of the season.

Serves 8 to 10

What's In It

- unsweetened flaked coconut (0.50 c.)
- Blueberries (1 c.) (0.50 c.)
- Coconut milk (2 tbsp.)
- Gluten free baking powder (1.50 tsp)
- Potato starch (0.33 c.)
- Brown rice flour (0.75 c.)
- Desiccated coconut (0.75 c. and 2 tbsp.)
- Free range eggs (2 large)

- Zest of lemon (1)
- Vanilla extract (1 tsp)
- Unrefined raw sugar (1 c.)
- Softened butter (0.50 c. and 1tbs)
- Gluten free icing sugar
- Softly whipped cream

How It's Made

- Preheat your oven to a temperature of 335 degrees f.
- Using a 9-inch round pan grease the pan with olive oil.
- Start by creaming sugar and butter until light and fluffy
- Stir in your vanilla and zest adding eggs, one at a time. Beating while adding eggs.
- Add desiccated coconut and sift it over the brown rice flour, the potato starch, and baking powder. Stir until

almost fully blended and then coconut milk and blueberries. Fold them together.

- Spoon your mix into a prepared tin, and place on top 0.50 cup of berries and flaked coconut.
- Place in oven and bake for 60 to 70 minutes till done, cool in pan.
- Using powdered sugar or coconut flour and sprinkle over the pan, serve with yoghurt.

Lemon-Honey and Thyme Sorbet

Makes about 600ml

What's In It

- Lemon juice (1.50 c.)
- Zest of lemons (2)
- Fresh thyme sprigs (small handful)
- Cold water (1 c.)
- Honey (0.75 c.- 1 c.)

How Its' Made

- Start with blending honey, with water, thyme sprigs, and lemon zest in a boiler and bring it to a boil, stirring to make sure it dissolves the honey.
- Boil for another minute then remove from the heat.
- Set it aside to cool.
- Strain your syrup into a jug and squeeze as much of the flavor as you can form your thyme leaves and zest, then toss them out.
- Mix in lemon juice to your syrup and chill at least 2 hours.
- Churn the mix into an ice cream machine, pour it into a bowl that is freezer proof.
- Freeze the ingredients for 1 hour, until your edges start to freeze. Then

beat with your hand mixer, mixing until smooth. Replace it in the freezer and repeat the process of blending 2 to 3 times. Let sit in the freezer and freeze for 2 hours.

Little Lemon and Lavender Cakes (Gluten Free)

This serves 6

What's In It

- Lemon juice, pure icing sugar, maqui powder (optional)
- Gluten free baking powder (2 tsp)
- Potato starch (2 tbsp.)
- Almond meal (0.50 c.)
- Brown rice Flour (0.75 c.)
- Dried lavender (1 tsp)
- Milk (2 tsp)
- Zest of lemon (1)
- Free range eggs (2 large)

- Blended unrefined raw sugar (0.50 c.)
- Butter (100 g)

How It's Made

- Heat your oven to a temperature of 335 degrees f. Using a small Bundt cake and olive oil spray for greasing it, prepare the pan.
- Melt butter over a low temperature, set it to the side for cooling
- Whisk some eggs and sugar with an electric beater for 5 to 8 minutes.
- It should be lovely and thickened.
- Next, add in some lemon zest and lavender.
- Using a sieve, place it over your rice flour and sieve the almond flour, baking powder, and potato starch.

- Add in the almond meal bits that don't go through the sieve and mix everything together.
- Fold it all together until it is half mixed.
- Next, add in some milk and the cooled butter, folding it together.
- Now, divide the mix evenly into cake tins, and bake for 20 minutes. The cakes should rise and be golden.
- Take it out of the oven and set to the side for 5 minutes, then transfer to a wire rack to cool.
- Now, mix your icing by combining icing sugar with lemon juice to get a desired consistency for icing.
- Using the maqui powder color the icing and then begin to drizzle it over the tops, the cakes should be cooled. Let a little drip down the side.

- Using extra lavender if you so like to decorate the tops.
- They can store for 2 to 3 days in an air tight container.

Gluten and Dairy Free Spiced Pear and Almond Cake Recipe

You can use olive oil in place of butter in this recipe. Using ground almonds will keep things form drying out. The pear slices add texture. If you want more ginger flavor you can add in a bit more crystallized ginger for flavor.

Serves 10 to 12

What's In It

- Pears (2 peeled)
- Sliced almonds (0.33 cup)
- Pure icing sugar for dusting
- Mixed spice (0.50 tsp)

- Sea salt (0.25 c.)
- Ginger (ground) (1 tsp)
- Cinnamon (ground) (1 tsp)
- Baking powder (1 tsp)
- Fine brown rice flour (0.33 c.)
- Almonds (ground) (2.75 c.)
- Extra virgin olive oil (0.33 C.)
- Lemon zest (1)
- Vanilla extract (1 tsp)
- Unrefined raw sugar (0.666 c.)
- Free range eggs (4 large)

How It's Made

- Start by heating your oven to 350 degrees f. Grease the baking sheet and place baking paper into the pan.
- Start by beating your eggs and vanilla extract, along with sugar using an electric mixer or beater.

Continue to beat the mix for 5 minutes until it is thick, and pale.
- Next, add lemon zest and sprinkle some olive oil in, continue to beat until all the ingredients are blended.
- Now, add in some almonds and sieve over some brown rice flour, spices, and baking powder.
- Then, gently fold with a large metal spoon until all ingredients are blended. Now fold in some pear slices, and then transfer to a cake pan. Toss some sliced almonds and bake the cake for 55 to 60 minutes.
- Take it out of the oven and cool it for 10 minutes then flip it onto a wire rack to cool until room temperature.
- Using the icing sugar dust, the cake and then serve it slightly warm.
- This can store for 3 days in an airtight container.

Roasted Quince and Cardamom Popsicles

For vegan popsicles use a dairy free yoghurt. To have yoghurt bowls reduce the sugar content since popsicles need more sugar.

Makes 6 to 8 servings

What's In It

- Natural plain yoghurt (dairy free) (0.50 c.)
- Cardamom pods (3)
- Filtered water (0.25 c. cold)
- Coconut sugar (0.25 c.)
- Roasted quince puree (2 c.)

How It's Made

- To prepare the quince puree you need 4 to 5 quinces that are halved lengthwise.

- Stat the oven on a temperature of 320 degrees f. Arrange the halves onto a baking sheet that has a little water in it and roast the quinces for 3.5 hours to 4 hours until they are deeply colorful and tender.
- Take it off of the heat and set to the side to cool. Scoop out the tender bits in the center of the flesh, discarding the seeds and the skin.
- Now you are left with the leather-like tops which are a delicious treat that is sweet and sour.
- Move the peeled quinces and jelly like roasting juices to a blender and blend until it is completely smooth.
- If you cannot get it super smooth, then use a sieve to weed out any lumps.
- Next start the other portion of the popsicle.

- First, add the sugar, water and cardamom into a boiler and bring it to a boil over medium to high heat, continue cooking while stirring and the sugar is dissolving.
- Turn your heat down to a simmer of 1 to 2 minutes, the water should be reduced by half.
- Take it off the heat and set it aside for 5 minutes, removing the cardamom pods and then add to the blender with the quince paste, yoghurt and a pinch of fine sea salt.
- Now, blend on high until it is smooth.
- Spoon the thickened mix into 6 to 8 popsicle molds and tap the mold to help it all settle, releasing the air bubbles. Now, insert a wooden stick and freeze them for 4 to 6 minutes or until they are frozen. Using warm

water rinse the molds to release the popsicles.

Gluten Free Honey Almond Cake with Pistachios, Strawberries and Hibiscus Rose Syrup

You can get dried hibiscus flowers at a local health food store. Using 1 to 2 tsp of flowers placed in the bottom of the mug. Pour your boiling water over and set aside to steep for 5 minutes. For lactose free use ghee instead of better and use a coconut based vanilla ice cream. This makes 4 to 6 servings.

What's In it

- Punnet strawberries (250 g)
- Vanilla ice cream (to serve)
- Free range egg (1 large)
- Vanilla extract (1 tsp)

- Milk or milk alternative (rice milk is ok) (0.25 c.)
- Gluten free baking powder (1.50 tsp)
- Gluten free corn flour (2 tbsp.)
- Brown rice flour (0.25 c.)
- Ground almonds (almond flour/almond meal) (0.75 c.)
- Honey (0.25 c.)
- Butter (Ghee) (75 g)

Hibiscus Rose Syrup

- Rose water (2 to 3 tsp)
- Unrefined raw sugar (0.33 c.)
- Brewed hibiscus tea (0.75 c.)

How it's Made

- Start by heating the oven to a temperature of 160c. Using Olive oil spray, thinly coat a baking pan. Then

line the pan with foil, until it hangs over the edge of the pan.
- Next, place some butter or ghee, along with honey in a boiler and heat at a low heat, the butter or ghee should be melted.
- Remove it from your heat and set it aside. Place some ground almonds into a bowl and sieve over some brown rice flour, corn flour and some baking powder.
- Whisking to blend the ingredients, thoroughly.
- In another bowl, whisk your milk, eggs, and vanilla together. Then pour it over the dry ingredients with the honey mix and the milk mix. Stirring until it is just blended.
- Pour the mix into the pan, making sure it evenly fills the pan. Scatter with some chopped pistachios.

- Place the pan in the oven and bake for 20 minutes, it should be lightly golden.
- Take it out of the oven and set it aside to cool at room temperature.
- Now, combine your hibiscus tea and your raw sugar into a medium boiler, bringing it to a boil over the temperature of medium to high heat. Continue stirring to ensure the sugar has melted fully before it boils. Once the boiler is boiling, turn the heat slightly down and simmer for 4 to 5 minutes or until reduced slightly and like syrup.
- Now, take it off of the heat and stir in your rose water.
- Pour it into a small jug.
- When serving, slice your honey cake into some squares or diamonds and place in a bowl. Using a handful of

- sliced strawberries, you can scoop ice cream on top.
- Sprinkle with extra chopped pistachios and some hibiscus rose syrup.
- The cake is best eaten the same day. It will store in an airtight container for 2 to 3 days. Hibiscus rose syrup can store in a glass jar for 5 days in the fridge.

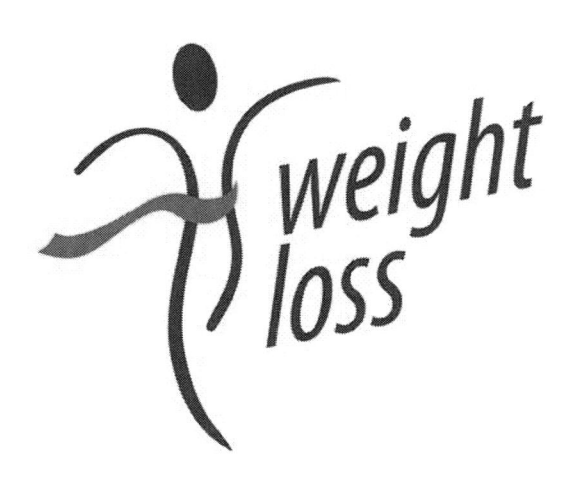

weight loss

Bonus Chapter: GERD Diet for Weight Loss

Bonus Chapter: GERD Diet for Weight Loss

There are several ways you can lose weight and help alleviate your GERD symptoms. There are seven tips to losing weight with GERD. Below I have listed those seven tips.

- **Eat smaller meals**-Your stomach is designed to expand based on how much you are putting into it. Once you stretch it too far, it can be damaged. So, eating smaller portions will not only help correct the stomach expansion but also allow you to begin a weight loss journey. You will also be able to alleviate your GERD by reducing the amount of food stored in your stomach at one time. The appropriate size for a small meal would be the size of your fist. This means that you should eat 3 small meals with 2 to 3 small healthy snacks a day or eat a small meal ever 2 to 2.5 hours. This helps keep your blood sugar under control and keeps you from getting hunger pains.

- **Eat fewer calories**- When you eat fewer calories your body will draw its energy form the fat that is being stored in your body. This helps to eliminate your excess fat that your body has been holding on to. Do not eat too many carbohydrates since they slow the process of burning fat. When we reduce our intake to a healthy level we are helping control our GERD. Each age group has a specific level of healthy intake of calories. So, knowing what is healthy for you is important.

- **Do not eat within three hours of bedtime**-this is one that many people struggle with. When we eat within three hours of bedtime we end up going to bed without our foods fully processed. This results in GERD symptoms and also causes us to hold on to excess fat. hours are the average time it takes for food to digest for an adult. That is why we suggest not eating within 3 hours of bedtime. This does depend on the type so foods you consume but most of them take 3 hours. It is 3 hours for half of your food to move to lower stomach and 5 hours for a full empty stomach. Another way to prevent GERD is to sleep on your left side as much as you can this helps the stomach wrap under the lung and keeps the food in a pocket, so you don't experience GERD symptoms.

- **Eat slowly**-No matter what you eat, just do it slowly. This helps you chew the food more thoroughly which improves your digestion and shortens your digestion cycle. Smaller pieces of food mean less acidic digestive juices are required for digestion. The other benefit of eating slower is that it gives you brain time to catch up to the fact that your stomach is getting full. If you have ever noticed that sometimes when you eat slow you eat less food? That is because your brain has time to catch up with the stomach processes.
- **Stay away from trigger foods.** Trigger foods are ones that trigger your GERD symptoms. Avoiding

acidic or acid producing foods is a great start. Most the time spicy foods or ones high in saturated fats and trans fat are triggers for GERD symptoms. You should also avoid coffee, tomatoes, tomato products, chocolate, alcohol, carbonated beverages, and excessive refined sugar. Sometimes citrus and mint needs to be avoided as well.

- **Eat helpful foods.** Try to incorporate some alkaline foods such as avocado, olives, bananas, and eggs. Limited amounts of cheese. These help to neutralize the acids in your stomach.
- **Walk after eating.** Taking a walk after eating will help with the digestive process. This will also help eliminate the GERD symptoms. It helps you to not lie down or over eat

because instead of being complacent after eating you are being active.

One great diet that works wonderfully with the GERD weight loss plan is the Mediterranean diet. In the Mediterranean diet works well for most people who are trying to not only loss weight but also eat more healthy foods. The Mediterranean diet has been found to reduce cardiovascular mortality, cancer, Alzheimer's disease, Parkinson's and over-all improvement son your health.

The benefits of the Mediterranean diet are;

- **Low in processed foods and sugar**- diet consist of foods and ingredients that very closely resemble nature and what is grown in nature. It includes olive oil, legumes, beans, fruits, vegetables, cereal products that are unrefined, small portion of animal products. There is low to no sugar intake and free of all GMO's such as high fructose corn syrup. The Mediterranean diet only uses honey and fruit for sweetener. Other than plants, you would eat locally caught fish and small portions of grass fed cows, goats, and pigs.

- **It helps you lose weight in a healthy way**-you lose weight without feeling hungry. You get to maintain your weight because the diet is sustainable. Most people find doing the Mediterranean diet worthwhile. It can be low-carb, low-protein, or one of the two. You can do a completely vegan form of the

Mediterranean diet or you can do a meat-eating form or a vegetarian form. It is versatile for all dietary differences

- **It can improve your heart health**- By following the Mediterranean diet as specified you can significantly reduce your mortality rates based on all health conditions, especially heart disease. A diet rich in alpha-linolenic acid has been proven to reduce cardiac death by 30% and sudden cardia death by 45%. Studies also show that consuming more olive oil will decrease blood pressure. It's also great for lowering hypertension because it makes nitric oxide more bioavailable, which keeps arteries dilated and clear. It also helps combat the disease promoting effects of oxidation.

- **Helps Fight Cancer**- Omega-6 and omega-3 essential fatty acids and high amount s of fiber, antioxidants, and polyphenols that are found in vegetables, fruits, olive oil and wine. Plant foods, fruits, and vegetables help fight cancer in every way. They provide antioxidants, protecting DNA from damage. It stops cell mutation and lowering inflammation which also aids in delaying tumor growth. Olive oil might even be a natural cure for cancer and reduces the risks of colon cancer and bowel cancers.
- **Prevents of Treats Diabetes**- a low sugar diet with lots of produce and fats can naturally lower diabetic issues and essentially cure diabetes.

- **Protects Cognitive Health and Can Improve Your Mood-** Mediterranean diet is a natural Parkinson's Disease treatment. It's a great way to preserve your memory. It is considered a step in the right direction for treating Alzheimer's.
- **Might Help You Live Longer-** High plant food diet and a healthy fats diet is guaranteed to increase the longevity of your life. Monosaturated Fat is about to lower levels of heart disease, depression, cancer, cognitive decline, inflammatory disease, and Alzheimer's disease.
- **Helps You De stress and relax-** chronic stress can kill your quality of life. It can increase your weight and destroy your health. The Mediterranean diet allows you to slow down and eat at a slower pace.

It allows for physical activity and increases your mood.

Here is an example of the Mediterranean diet:

Fennel Apple Soup Recipe

This meal is gluten free, paleo, and great as a main course or side dish.

It serves 2 to 4 people and takes 30 minutes.

What's In It

- Thyme sprigs (2 to 3)
- Chicken broth (1 quart)
- Apples (2 large, peeled, cored and diced)
- Fennel Bulbs (stems removed and diced) (2 medium)
- Onion (chopped) (1)

- Coconut oil (2 tbsp.)

How it's Made

- Start with heating your coconut in a boiler.
- Sauté your onions over low temperature for 10 to 15 minutes, until they are almost brown.
- Next, add some fennel and Apples to the boiler. Then cook for 5 to 10 minutes until softened or browned.
- Now, add chicken stock and thyme.
- Once everything is prepared, puree the soup in the blender; it should be smooth and creamy.
- Serve and enjoy!

So how do you start the Mediterranean Diet?

How can you incorporate the Mediterranean diet into your lifestyle?

What steps can you take to implement this diet plan? In this next section, we will discuss how we can incorporate the Mediterranean diet into our life and what it takes to start losing weight with the Mediterranean diet.

- You can eat lots of vegetables.
- Always eat breakfast.
- Eat seafood twice a week.
- Cook a vegetarian meal one night a week.
- Enjoy dairy products in moderation.
- For dessert, eat fresh fruit.
- Use good fats.
- Quick start to a Mediterranean diet:
- Sautéing food in olive oil instead of butter.
- Eating more fruits and vegetables by eating salads as entrée, starter or side dish.

- Only snacking on fruits.
- Adding vegetables to other dishes.
- Chose whole grains.
- Substitute fish for red meat, twice a week.
- Limit your high fat dairy, use only 1% or 2% milk.
- Use carrots, celery, broccoli and salsa.
- Quinoa with stir fried vegetables.
- Sandwich fillings in whole wheat tortillas.
- Pudding made with skim or 1% milk.

CHAPTER SUMMARY:

11.1. In this chapter, we talked about the Mediterranean diet and how it can help you with your GERD treatment. There are several diets plans out there, however, the Mediterranean diet is one of the best for helping cure illness and disease. We discuss how the Mediterranean diet helps you lose weight when having GERD.

11.2. Next, we discuss the benefits of the Mediterranean diet and how it does benefit you. We discuss the conditions that it can help improve cure and why. We talk about what Doctors say about the Mediterranean diet and the benefits they have seen.

11.3. The last section we discuss one example of a Mediterranean diet meal recipe. The Fennel Apple Soup Recipe is a great recipe that is hearty and full of good nutrients which helps keep you healthy longer.

YOUR QUICK START ACTION STEP:

11.4. How can you implement the Mediterranean diet into your lifestyle? This is simple. Start by swapping out your food options to a healthier option.

- Chose whole grains.
- Substitute fish for red meat, twice a week.
- Limit your high fat dairy, use only 1% or 2% milk.
- Use carrots, celery, broccoli and salsa.
- Quinoa with stir fried vegetables.
- Sandwich fillings in whole wheat tortillas.
- Pudding made with skim or 1% milk.

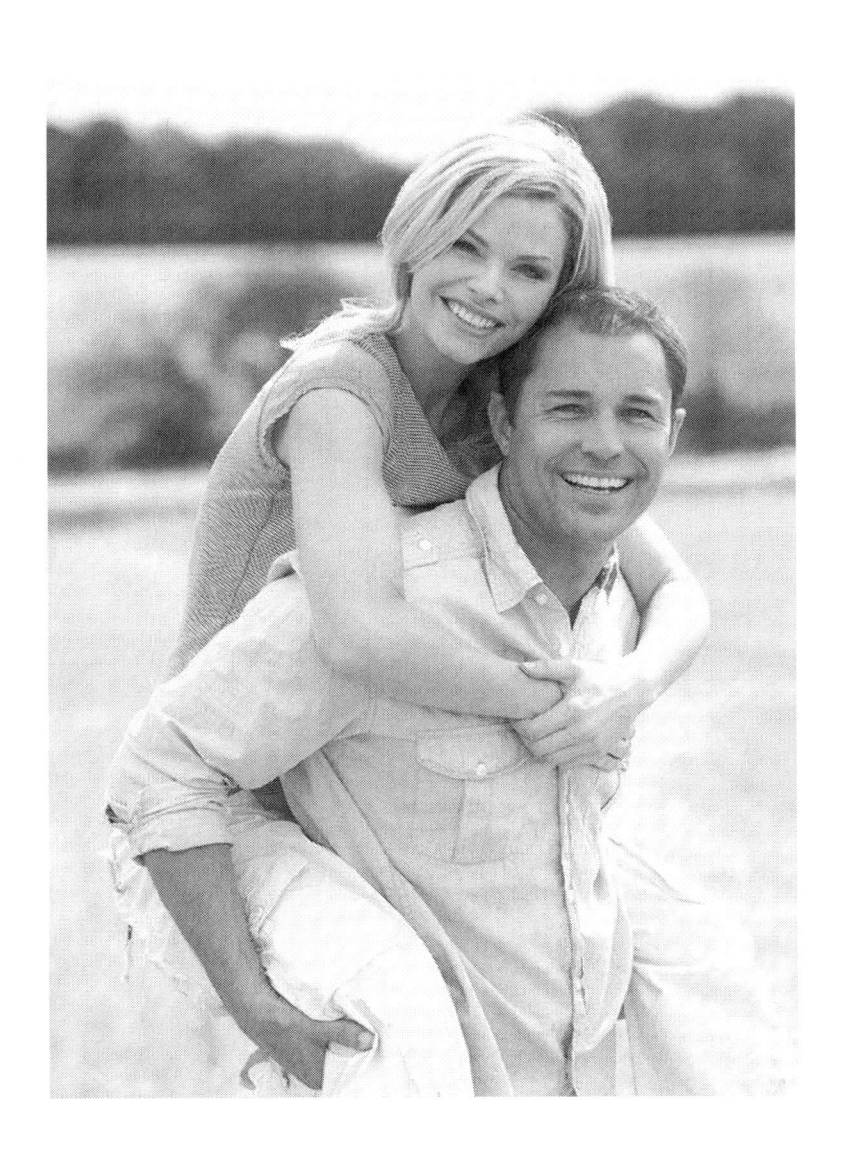

Conclusion

I hope this book was able to help you to heal your GERD symptoms with the recipes in this book and the natural remedies that are effective and proven to work.

The next step is to start using the tools outlined in the quickstep actions to help build a GERD Diet Meal Plan. All of the recipes in this book are designed to give you a starting point for building your dietary meal plan. Once you start changing your dietary plan you can start changing your life. GERD is a painful condition that can last for many years without proper a proper diet. If you eat right and use natural remedies you can reverse the damage that GERD has caused as well as stop the current symptoms.

Finally, if this book has given you value and helped you in any way, then I'd like to ask you for a favor if you would be kind enough to leave a review for this book on Amazon? It'd be greatly appreciated!

Thank you and good luck!

Printed in Poland
by Amazon Fulfillment
Poland Sp. z o.o., Wrocław